PTCB Exam Prep 2023-2024

Updated Study Guide + 540 Test Questions and Detailed Answer Explanations for the Pharmacy Technician Certification Exam (6 Full-Length Practice PTCE Tests)

Printed in the United States of America

Table of Contents

Introduction

Pharmacy technicians are indispensable members of the pharmaceutical and drug delivery workforce. As the baby boomers age, the need for prescription medicine increases. This trend has exponentially increased the need for pharmacists, pharmacy technicians and other pharmaceutical professionals.

Functions of a Certified Pharmacy Technician

Prescription processing

This includes filling patient prescriptions; labeling them; educating patients on the route, mode of action, side effects, interactions and contraindications of their drugs; maintaining the drug inventory; setting up bills and more.

Dispensary

This includes compounding of ointment creams, oral solutions and large amounts of IV drugs; packaging of bulk drugs; preparing IV drugs for administration; preparing chemotherapeutic drugs, etc.

Collaboration

Apart from working under the supervision of a pharmacist, a pharmacy technician collaborates with other professionals, such as members of the clinical team, including doctors, registered nurses, nursing practitioners, physician assistants, etc., and nonclinical members, like insurance companies, pharmaceutical companies, drug reps and so on. The pharmacy technician can also collaborate with community members, caregivers, patients' families, etc.

Patient education

Pharmacy technicians educate patients on the pharmacodynamics and pharmacokinetics of the drugs in a prescription, including side effects, dose, route of administration, indications, contraindications, etc.

How to Become a Certified Pharmacy Technician

Education requirements

Obtain a high school diploma or GED equivalent – Successful pharmacy technicians usually have a background in biology, chemistry, physics and mathematics.

Take an accredited pharmacy technician course – This can be from a college, a technical school, a distance learning program or a compulsory training course given by companies.

College programs – Colleges offer two- and four-year programs. Most technicians prefer the two-year programs. Students who have a BSc degree with a major in science courses like biology or chemistry can go on to take two-year diploma programs. All in all, a student's choice to enroll in a two- or four-year program depends on individual factors. College programs are quite intense, with scheduled classes, seminars and laboratory or clinic work.

One benefit of choosing a college degree is that your certificate is universally recognized and accepted. This makes it easy for you to switch to another career when you wish to. Another benefit is the ability to further your education. However, college/diploma programs are expensive and require a time commitment. Community colleges are good considerations if you want to cut down on cost, commute from home and work as you go to school.

Technical school program – This option is suitable for people who do not have sufficient time or finances for college/diploma programs. Technical schools offer training in specific areas, with lots of hands-on training. However, coursework is not as extensive as that of college programs. The duration of learning is significantly shorter than college programs, ranging from about eight to 18 months.

Proprietary training program – This includes mandatory programs offered by employers/companies to their new employees and staff. Hospitals, large retail pharmacy stores and other health-care providers provide training programs to entry-level pharmacy technicians.

Distance learning program – This type of program is taught online. It is convenient for people who want to keep their day jobs and earn their degrees on the side. Courses are taught on a platform on the internet, and the curriculum is often self-paced. A downside to this method is its unsuitability for people who are not self-motivated. Distance learning programs are not as resource intensive as traditional college programs.

Get certified

Certification is given by regional bodies after candidates successfully pass the required exams. In the United States, 45 states make certification mandatory for licensure. Certification can be obtained from the National Healthcareer Association (NHA) or the Pharmacy Technician Certification Board (PTCB). After passing the exams, successful candidates are awarded the title of certified pharmacy technician (CPhT). All necessary information about the certification exam conducted by the PTCB will be discussed in this book.

The CPhT is an entry certificate. Pharmacy technicians can decide to deepen their knowledge by obtaining additional certifications in nuclear pharmacy tech (NPT), chemotherapy or sterile products.

Recertification

Recertification is done every two years for both the NHA and the PTCB. The NHA requires 10 hours of continuing education, while the PTCB requires 20 hours.

Career Options

Retail pharmacy technicians – These professionals make up 70% of the workforce of pharmacy technicians. They work in retail stores, dispensing drugs, forwarding prescription claims to insurance companies, managing billing and transactions and processing prescriptions.

Hospital pharmacy technicians – These technicians work in hospitals. Just like retail technicians, they also fill medication orders, process prescriptions, pre-package drugs, educate patients and evaluate drugs and adherence. These professionals have extensive training.

Rehabilitation center pharmacy technicians – These professionals work in private establishments and pharmacies located in rehab facilities. They attend to patients with mental health disorders and substance abuse disorders, and they collaborate with rehabilitation specialists.

Community pharmacy technicians – These professionals work in community settings. They assist pharmacists in attending to patients onsite or via phone. They manage drug inventories, pre-package drugs, educate patients and complete daily administrative tasks.

Central pharmacy operations technicians – These professionals work in central fill centers, managing drug inventories organizing pharmaceutical products and labeling shelves. They have extensive knowledge of pharmacy operations.

Government agencies – Pharmacy technicians are found at all levels of government. They can work in the armed forces, Veterans Administration, Federal Bureau of Prisons, Prison Health Service and more. They work under the supervision of pharmacists, taking drug inventories, processing prescription orders and performing administrative tasks. Although this career option does not guarantee opportunities for career growth, it offers job security.

Managed care – Here, pharmacy technicians work with pharmacy benefit companies and health insurance companies. They review authorization requests and drug claims, educate patients, offer various pharmacy services and collaborate with health-care providers, case managers and others to ensure an efficient continuum of care.

Nuclear pharmacy – This specialty is focused on the safe creation, packaging and transportation of radioactive drugs. It is a highly specialized field and requires extensive training. Pharmacy technicians are trained to calculate, compound and label radioactive drugs, manage inventories and package and transport drugs safely.

Remuneration

The median annual earnings for CPhTs is $35,100, with a range of $25,400 to $50,430. Earnings are projected to rise as demand for more CPhTs increases over the decade. Factors that affect earnings include:

Location

According to the Bureau of Labor Statistics, the top CPhT earners are in Washington (annual earnings $42,390), Oregon ($41,160), California ($40,120), the District of Columbia ($39,930) and Alaska ($35,190). These areas have positions for CPhTs in universities, federal institutions and outpatient facilities. However, before CPhTs consider switching locations to increase their earnings, they should consider the impact of food, housing and taxes on income.

Employers

Generally, public establishments pay more than private establishments. CPhTs who work in federal institutions, colleges and outpatient care facilities earn the highest salaries. CPhTs who work in retail stores earn the lowest.

Work experience

Generally, more experienced CPhTs earn more than their junior colleagues. CPhTs in the top level earn an average of $41,790 yearly. These people make up the 90th percentile. Senior-level CPhTs earn an average of $35,542. They make up the 75th percentile. Mid-level CPhTs earn an average of $29,690. They are found in the 50th percentile. Junior-level CPhTs, who are in the 25th percentile, earn an average of $24,801. Lastly, entry-level CPhTs earn an average of $21,093. They are found in the 10th percentile.

Traits of a Successful Pharmacy Technician

Attention to detail

Successful CPhTs pay attention to detail. They guarantee the safety of their patients by accurately measuring, calculating and mixing drugs, dispensing the right doses, updating patients' drug information and filling prescription orders.

Pharmaceutical literacy

Successful CPhTs are knowledgeable about pharmaceutical terminology and literature, including medical terms. Apart from this, they can communicate this knowledge to their patients using simple terms.

Communication skills

A CPhT knows how to communicate. Communication is two-way—knowing how to speak and knowing how to listen. Skill in these two aspects is crucial. This is because the CPhT spends time communicating with patients, health-care providers, caregivers and communities.

Social skills

A successful CPhT must know how to collaborate with other members of the health team and patients, including families and caregivers.

Pros and Cons of Becoming a CPhT

Pros

Lucrativeness

The role of a CPhT is a lucrative one. There are over 400,000 CPhTs in the United States. This figure is projected to increase by 12% over the decade as the adult population ages, lives longer and needs drug interventions for chronic diseases.

Flexibility in career trajectory

Because of the inter-relationship between pharmacy and other health fields, a CPhT can switch career paths. For example, a CPhT with a diploma or associate degree in pharmacy technology can go on to become a registered nurse, a nursing assistant, a certified phlebotomist, etc. More ambitious CPhTs can switch to become pharmacists, physician assistants, medical doctors, etc.

Cons

Burnout
Mental and physical burnout is a factor to consider for CPhTs who spend a lot of time calculating and standing, hunched over desks or laptops. Also, the calculations and administrative tasks can become monotonous and tedious.

Hazards
Like other health-care providers, CPhTs are vulnerable to health hazards in the form of biological hazards (such as during IV drug administration).

Differences Between a Pharmacist and a CPhT

Education

Pharmacists have more extensive coursework and training than CPhTs. While CPhTs spend an average of two years training to earn their degree, pharmacists spend six to eight years. They start with foundational courses like math, biology and chemistry in the first two years and then progress to advanced courses like physiology, molecular pharmacology, pharmacy management, pharmacy practice, medicinal biochemistry and therapeutics in the last four years.

If students with BSc degrees in other fields wish to become pharmacists, they spend four years obtaining a doctoral degree (PharmD). After six years of study, one year is used for an internship training program.

Certification

Certification for CPhTs is awarded by the PTCB. This board administers the Pharmacy Technician Certification Exam (PTCE). Another exam is the Ex Certified Pharmacy Technician (ExCPT) exam given by the NHA. Either one of these certifying exams is required.

Pharmacists must take two exams for certification. The first is the North American Pharmacist Licensure Exam (NAPLEX), while the second is a state jurisprudence exam or the Multistate Pharmacy Jurisprudence Exam (MPJE).

Remuneration

Pharmacists earn more than CPhTs. The average salary of a CPhT is $35,100, while that of a pharmacist is $128,710.

However, because more people are getting their prescriptions online, the role of pharmacists is projected to eventually decline by 2%, while that of CPhTs is projected to increase by 4%.

Scope of practice

A pharmacist is licensed to carry out drug consultations with patients, physicians and other health-care providers. CPhTs are not licensed to do so. Furthermore, CPhTs cannot work without supervision from pharmacists.

Chapter 1: The PTCE

The Pharmacy Technician Certification Exam (PTCE) is the gold standard for certifying CPhTs. It is also the most popular exam used in certifying CPhTs in the United States and Canada. This exam is created and administered by the PTCB, an NGO that offers certification exams for CPhTs.

Since 1995, the PTCB has been committed to certifying technicians who can guarantee the safety of the public. To do this, the PTCB uses a set of formulated and standardized cognitive tests that can verify the proficiency of technicians in the United States, the District of Columbia and all the US territories. Apart from administering certification exams, the PTCB provides resources for ongoing and continuous learning and encourages collaboration among board members and employer-employee relationships via employer resources and programs. It also provides other resources that encourage learning and growth for all technicians. The PTCB prides itself on its ability to provide services that are diverse, nondiscriminatory and inclusive.

The PTCE exams provided by the PTCB are accredited by the National Commission for Certifying Agencies (NCCA) and recognized by pharmacy associations in individual states, as well as the American Pharmacists Association, the National Association of Boards of Pharmacy and the Society of Health-System Pharmacists. This accreditation and recognition means that the PTCB has met all the requisite requirements in developing, implementing and maintaining its certification exam.

Eligibility Requirements

Training

There are two pathways for meeting the training requirement.

Pathway 1 – This involves completing education via an accredited training program. There are over 1,400 programs listed on the PTCB website.

Pathway 2 – This involves a work experience of at least 500 hours as a CPhT. This pathway is useful for experienced candidates who were not able to attend an educational program.

Character

Before starting the application process, candidates are screened for moral behavior. Screening questions assess if candidates have had a revocation, suspension or relinquishment of their licenses; if they have been fired by an employer or supervisor for dishonest behavior; if they have been convicted of felonies; if they have been arrested for violating laws concerning possession of alcohol and drugs or sexual assault; and if they have been offered immunity by a grand jury.

How to Register for the Exam

Application

Application is done solely online at https://www.ptcb.org/credentials/certified-pharmacy-technician.

You can apply to take the exam by following these steps:

Create a profile

This stage is required for new users. Previous users can log in using their usernames and passwords. Remember to use a valid email address.

Fill out the application form

Make sure that you meet the requirements for eligibility by filling in the required information as instructed.

Upload documents

Upload scanned copies of your certifications of completion of the education program or work training. The certificate should include your official name, the title of the training program/education and the date of completion. Also upload your diploma certificates or unofficial transcripts where applicable, along with an official letter from the program establishment or training provider. This letter should have a letterhead and include your official name, date of completion and title of program/education.

Payment

Payment is made during the application and is only accepted in USD by credit card or debit card. Personal checks, money orders and company checks are not acceptable. The application and exam fee cost $129. Payment can be made by employers/educators through the direct billing method. The billing options available are vouchers, tokens, IP address identification and preapprovals.

Notification of eligibility status

You will be notified via email of your eligibility to take the exam within 30 days of your application. This eligibility is valid for 90 days. If you are in the Assessment-Based Certificate Program, you have two 90-day windows to schedule the exam. You must reschedule your exam to the next test window before the first window expires.

Withdrawal from exams

If you wish to withdraw from the exam, notify the PTCB at least a day before the end of the authorization to test (ATT) window. After withdrawal, refunds will be made three to four weeks later, in the same format the application fee was paid. An administrative fee of $25 will be deducted.

Authorization to test

If you have completed your application, paid the required application fees and had your application forms verified and approved, you will be given an ATT. This ATT is sent via email. You can print the ATT and read the instructions on how to schedule exams via Pearson VUE, the computer-based testing partner. Please review the ATT slip for accuracy and consistency because your name must match your name on the primary and secondary ID.

A time frame (90 days) to take the exam is written on the ATT. If you fail to take the exam during this time frame and do not withdraw or reschedule the exam, you are automatically ineligible for the exam and must apply again.

Scheduling an Exam

To schedule your exam, read the instructions on the ATT. Scheduling is done on the Pearson VUE website. On the website, first-time exam takers are required to create an account. To schedule the exam, use the ID number on the notification email. After scheduling the exam, Pearson VUE will send a notification email that confirms the scheduled test date and time, including phone numbers and the address of the test center and the directions to the test venue. Reservations are made on a first-come, first-served basis.

Rescheduling/Canceling the Exam

If you wish to reschedule or cancel your exam within your approved test window, you are free to do so as long as rescheduling is done within the 90-day window and at least 24 business hours before the scheduled exam. If you fail to reschedule and do not show up for the exam, you will be recognized as a no-show.

You are also free to request an emergency withdrawal if there is an emergency on the exam day. Events categorized as emergencies by the PTCB include serious accidents, serious injuries, illnesses, unexpected admissions in hospitals, a court appearance and the death of an immediate family member. If any of these occur, you should fill out and submit the Emergency Withdrawal Request Form and upload an official document (police report, medical report, obituary, etc.) that attests to the emergency. These documents must be sent to the PTCB at least 48 hours before the end of your ATT window. If the emergency withdrawal is approved, a full refund will be made in two to three weeks.

No-Show Policy

If you fail to reschedule your exam at least 24 business hours before the test date and fail to show up for the test, you will be considered a no-show and will forfeit the fee.

Retake Policies

If you are unsuccessful on the first exam attempt, you must wait 60 days before a second attempt. If you are unsuccessful the second time, you must wait another 60 days before making a third attempt. If you are unsuccessful a third time, you must wait six months before making a fourth attempt. After four attempts, you must complete preparation activities and show evidence to the PTCB for review. If the evidence is approved, you can then make additional attempts at passing the exam.

There are no limits to the number of attempts you can make to pass the test, but each attempt requires a new application and fees. You are encouraged to prepare adequately for the exam. Preparation activities accepted by the PTCB include:

1. At least six months of tutoring by a PharmD or PTCB CPhT
2. Completed nonaccredited programs or review courses
3. Earning a CPhT associate degree (A.S.)

Recertification

PTCB CPhTs must renew their certification every five years. Renewal is done via documentation of at least 20 hours of continuing education. Applications for certification renewal commence 60 days before the end of the certificate's expiration. Professionals who do not renew their certification by this time must apply for reinstatement.

The 20 hours of continuing education (CE) must include at least an hour's worth of education each in pharmacy law and patient safety. CE hours must cover the core subjects and topic areas in the PTCE content outline or cover topics offered by providers accredited by the ACPE. Topics offered by these providers are designated as "T," meaning the topics are targeted toward CPhTs.

Reinstatement

Professionals who want to be reinstated into the PTCB must meet all recertification requirements and complete at least an hour of continuing education in pharmacy law.

Fees

Recertification costs $49, and reinstatement fees are $89. Late processing for recertification incurs an additional fee of $25, while requests for reprocessing incur an additional fee of $10.

What to Expect on the Exam Day

What to do

Check-in

You should arrive at the designated testing center at least 15 to 30 minutes before your scheduled time. This is to enable you to verify your identity during recheck, locate your seat and be comfortably settled before the exam begins. If you arrive more than 15 minutes after the exam, you will not be allowed to test. Items that are prohibited from the testing center include reference materials like books, papers and dictionaries and personal items like purses, headwear, hoodies, veils, coats, briefcases and more. Pearson VUE and the PTCB will not take responsibility for any missing or stolen items, so these items should be left at home or in a vehicle.

Identification

You must present two forms of identification. The primary identification should have your full name, photo and signature. Accepted forms are passports, green cards, driver's licenses, state identification cards, national identity cards and permanent resident cards. Your identification must have your name and signature. Examples are Social Security cards, credit cards, employment cards and student cards.

Temporary identification is not acceptable. If your name in the eligibility letter differs from the name on your identification, you must show proof of a name change (court order, divorce papers or marriage license).

If you do not have an approved identification, you will not be allowed to take the exam. You will be seen to have missed your appointment, and no refunds will be made. Before the exam begins, you are expected to confirm your name and the nature of the exam and must agree to the rules and regulations of Pearson VUE and the PTCB.

Mode of Exam Delivery

The PTCE exams are computer-based and administered via a testing facility. You will be assigned to your seat and computer by a test administrator. For security, you must show your approved ID cards. These cards will be verified by a security system. Also, you will be asked to sign to show attendance and have your photo taken. A palm vein biometric will also be collected. Video and audio recordings of the exam will be made.

Exam length

The exam lasts for two hours and has 90 multiple-choice questions, of which 10 are pretest items. You will not be able to distinguish test items from pretest items. You are expected to attempt all questions because there is no negative scoring for incorrect answers. The exam session is divided into a five-minute introduction to teach you how to interact with the interface; the exam itself, which lasts for 110 minutes; and five minutes for a survey.

Exam breaks

Test breaks are not allowed during the exam. Unscheduled breaks are taken on your own time, including security checks when you leave and re-enter the testing facility. You are expected to attempt all questions during the allotted time.

Test Accommodations

If you require testing accommodations, you must affirm your needs in the checkbox of your application form, download the Accommodation Request Form, fill it out and upload it with documents supporting your diagnosis. These documents should be approved by the appropriate health professional and must be submitted within 30 days of your notification of eligibility to take the exam.

Accommodation resources do not cost extra. Resources provided by the PTCB include an extension of testing time, recorders, readers, separate room and increased font size. You are not allowed to bring your own interpreters, recorders or readers.

Rules and Regulations

Testing facilities

1. You are not allowed to discuss or communicate verbally or in other formats with other test takers once they enter the examination hall.
2. You are not permitted to copy, duplicate, communicate or transmit the test content for any reason. Copying and duplicating test content is a violation of Pearson VUE's security policy. If you do any of these, you are at risk of being disqualified from the exam and may be reported to the PTCB and security officials.
3. Electronic devices of any kind are banned from the exam hall.
4. Personal items and effects are banned from the exam hall. These items should be stored in a safe place before admission into the hall. Pearson VUE is not liable for any missing or stolen property.
5. Abusive behavior toward the staff is prohibited. You are expected to be courteous, professional and respectful of the staff and the rules and regulations of the exam. If you are abusive to the staff, you are at risk of forfeiting the exam and being reported to the PTCB and security personnel.
6. Third parties are prohibited from entering the examination room.
7. You are prohibited from leaving the building or using telephones during the examination.
8. You are not allowed breaks during the exam.

Lateness/absence

You must be present on or before the time stated on the ATT. If you arrive late, you will not be allowed to take the exam. If you are absent on the exam day, you will be deemed ineligible. If you wish to take the exam, you must reapply.

Weather

Pearson VUE has the sole right to determine if weather or other circumstances can close the test center. If this happens, the exam may be rescheduled, and affected candidates will be sent an email for the rescheduled date. There will be no extra charges. The PTCB is not liable for any extra expenses caused by a test cancellation.

Clothes

You are advised to wear comfortable clothing suitable for an exam environment. If you have glasses, accessories and/or layered clothing, they will be inspected before you enter the exam hall.

Lockers

Lockers are available for you to store your personal effects. You should store these items before entering the exam hall. The PTCB cannot be held liable for missing or stolen items. If you have prohibited items, you will be automatically disqualified from the exam. The PTCB is at liberty to confiscate prohibited items.

Prohibited items

Prohibited items include bags, backpacks, cell phones, electronics, food, beverages, books, paper, tobacco, cigarettes, sunglasses, headphones, Bluetooth speakers, earpieces, large pieces of jewelry, watches, etc.

How the Exam Is Developed

The PTCB exam consists of four domains and 26 subdomains. To create the test, research is done on current principles and practices in the core domains of pharmacy technology. Data is collected from professionals, employers and educators.

After collation, the data is analyzed and results are used as a guide in creating test items. Experts in pharmacy technology are hired as members of the examination committee. These experts are from diverse geographical, practice and demographic regions in the United States. Experts are also hired based on clinical experience, qualifications and skills. They are then trained in the principles of writing test questions. Reviewers assess the test items on reliability, discrimination level, difficulty and performance.

Finally, members of the content team are responsible for creating and updating competent statements and test outlines, reviewing data from completed exams, evaluating test items created by item writers, approving the exam forms used on the test day and reviewing test items in item banks.

How Exams Are Scored

The Modified Angoff method is used to determine passing standards. This passing standard is based on a set of criteria created by the board of directors of the PTCB after consultations with psychometric experts and other professionals. This criterion-referenced method is based on minimum education, training and competence for entry-level technicians.

For this to happen, a minimum level of competence is established after consulting and collaborating with professionals from different areas of geographic backgrounds, expertise and areas of practice. Passing scores are scaled down to adjust for difficulty and variation of test items.

Getting Test Results

Results are given as pass/fail. Unofficial results are shown on the screen after completion of the exam. Official results are sent to your dashboard one to three weeks after the exam, along with certificates and wallet cards. Results are not given over the phone or via fax. Successful candidates can request that a copy of the results or scores be mailed to them.

Tips on How to Pass the PTCE

Passing the PTCE requires a combination of preparation, organization and mental attitude. Adequate preparation has a lot to do with the type of resource materials you prepare with, the amount of time you spend preparing and the capacity of your recall.

How to choose the right resource materials

Here are a few things to consider before choosing the right study materials for your exams.

Relevance

Your study materials should be relevant to the exam. To increase your chances of selecting relevant study materials, you can buy resources recommended by your tutors, colleagues and peers who have passed the exams.

Revised

The PTCB reviews the PTCE periodically. Therefore, your study materials should be current, updated and revised to reflect the standard.

Cost

Good resource materials do not need to be expensive. There are affordably priced study materials, such as this guide.

Highlights

Your study material should provide highlights on the distribution of test questions and priority areas to focus on. Focused concentration is a characteristic of effective studying. It is not possible or advisable to read broad and wide. The right study material should help you narrow your reading to specific and key areas.

Comprehensive rationales

Your study material should give comprehensive rationales to test questions and their answers. This fine-tunes your critical thinking and helps you identify subtle words and distinctions you did not notice before.

Organized

Your study material should be organized methodically. Study materials that break down complex content into outlines and sections improve recall. Disorganized study materials can slow down your preparation process.

How much time should you spend studying?

The answer depends on you. There is no one-size-fits-all study duration. But there are a few basic factors that can help you choose what is right for you.

Start early

Early preparation increases your chances of success because you have time to prepare, experiment and make mistakes. Yes, you can make mistakes in your studying, especially if you are taking the exam for the first time. You can use the wrong resource materials, and your study plan can be inefficient. Whatever the error, early preparation gives you room to adjust your study plan.

Have a study goal

Although your goal is to pass your exam, you will need a study goal to help you achieve this. Remember, your goal must be SMART: Specific, Measurable, Achievable, Relevant and Time-bound.

For example, let's say you have a study goal to review the 540 questions in this book in a month. This goal has met three requirements of the SMART goal. It is specific, measurable and time-bound. You will then have to assess if the goal is attainable. To do so, you will have to determine how many questions you can answer in a day, how much time will be allotted to each study session and if the amount of time you have allocated is feasible.

Create a study timetable

A study timetable assesses your steps to achieving your study goal. For example, let's say you have assessed the feasibility of reviewing this book's questions in one month. Your next step will be to create a detailed study timetable that shows how much time is allocated to each study session. A study plan helps you track your progress and keeps you disciplined and focused.

Choose the suitable study method

You should be familiar with your preferred study method and stick to it. There is no need to experiment with various learning methods because doing so may slow you down and deter you from hitting your target. For example, students always ask if they should study alone or in a group. Group studying has its advantages and disadvantages, and so does studying solo. The truth is that neither study method is better than the other. Some candidates study more efficiently on their own; some do better in groups. A good tip is to use both forms of study, devoting more time to your dominant study method. That way, you can harness the benefits of both.

Extracurricular activities

You should factor rest, sleep, breaks and physical activity into your study timetable. If you begin your studies on time, you will have enough time to rest and recharge before the exam.

How to improve your recall

Recall is an important aspect of studying. After all, what is the point of studying if you cannot recall significant information when you need to? Here are a few tips to improve your recall.

Read actively

As much as possible, try to engage your mind in the text. Here are a few tips to help you read actively:

Read with a Focus – This is where study and resource materials come in handy. By giving you areas to focus on, study materials increase your engagement and concentration.

Take Notes as You Read – As you read, you can make notes, create mnemonics, create questions or create a post-reading to-do list. You can also highlight sections that are significant to you.

Take Breaks – Active reading requires focus and effort, and if done correctly, it cannot be done over a long period. For example, it is advised that study sessions be kept to a range of two to three hours. Anything longer, and you may struggle to concentrate. At this point, you can take short breaks for power naps, hydration and refueling.

Study in a group

Group study can improve recall because it is an effective form of active reading. Group study is great for reviewing large numbers of test questions.

Use mnemonics

Mnemonics are great tools for improving your recall. However, use them only after you understand the concepts of the topic. Mnemonics include but are not limited to acronyms, rhymes, imagery, chunking and the use of loci.

Understand first principles

Pharmacy is a science that is based on the principles of fact, logic and reasoning. Understanding topics from a first-principle basis improves your ability to store and retrieve information. When studying, always try to link the information together, building on your knowledge methodically.

Sleep

Sleep consolidates short-term memory. An adult requires an average of seven to nine hours of sleep a night. Therefore, when you create your study plan, factor in your need for adequate sleep.

How to be organized

To increase your chances of success, you should organize your activities before and during the exam.

Early registration

We covered the importance of early registration in the previous chapter. It increases your chances of success because it switches you into study mode sooner. Early registration also helps you be prepared for unforeseen circumstances.

Punctuality

You should show up at your exam center at least 30 minutes early. This gives you time to verify your identity, acquaint yourself with the rules of the examination and adjust to the testing center environment.

Dressing
Aim to dress comfortably and professionally. Do not wear clothes that will draw unnecessary attention or slow you down. For example, coats are not allowed into the exam hall. If you get cold easily, do not wear clothes made of thin fabric.

Having the right mental attitude

A positive mental attitude is important for taking the exam, particularly if you are retaking it. Here are a few tips to boost a positive mental attitude.

Study group peers
You can get support from study group peers who share your goal.

Tutors and mentors
You can also get support and encouragement from your tutors and mentors.

Successful candidates
Successful candidates not only give you practical information and insight to help you succeed, they boost your confidence in passing the exam by giving you practical firsthand counsel.

Visualization and affirmation
Visualization and affirmation can boost your confidence and improve your attitude toward the exam.

Sleep
Adequate rest can improve your mood, attitude and cognitive function.

Chapter 2: Medications

This makes up 40% of the test content. Topic areas include:

Generic Names, Brand Names and Classifications of Medications

Drug nomenclature

This is a systematic method for naming drugs. It includes the generic name, chemical name and trade name.

Chemical name

The chemical name is also known as the scientific name. In this system of naming, drugs are named according to how the drug's molecules are structured. The most important chemical naming system for drugs is the International Union of Pure and Applied Chemistry (IUPAC) naming system. Chemical names are long and often difficult to remember. They are not used in conventional language. For example, the chemical name for propanol, a beta-blocker, is 1-(isopropylamino)-3-(1-naphthyloxy) propan-2-ol.

Examples of chemical names of popular drugs include:

N-acetyl-p-aminophenol – Acetaminophen

(RS)-2-(4-(2-methylpropyl)phenyl)propanoic acid – Ibuprofen

ethyl 4-(8-chloro-5,6-dihydro-11H-benzo[5,6]cyclohepta[1,2-b]pyridin-11-ylidene) -1-piperidinecarboxylate – Loratadine

(3R,5R)-7-[2-(4-fluorophenyl)-3-phenyl-4-(phenylcarbamoyl)-5-propan-2-ylpyrrol-1-yl]-3,5-dihydroxyheptanoic acid – Atorvastatin

Generic names

Generic names are used for drug groups with similar actions. They are useful in identifying the class of a drug and its active ingredient. They are used for drug labels, prescription forms, advertisements, clinical trials, drug trials, research and scientific journals. Generic names are also called nonproprietary names. When a drug passes development, tests and regulations, the pharmaceutical company then gives it a trade name.

The International Nonproprietary Name (INN) system was created by the World Health Organization in 1953. Other bodies—like the Australian Approved Name (AAN) system, the United States Adopted Name (USAN) system, the British Approved Name (BAN) system and the Japanese Accepted Name (JAN) system—have their own systems for conferring generic names on drugs.

Examples of generic names

Stem	Drug class	Example
-cillin	Penicillin antibiotics	oxacillin, carbenicillin, penicillin, amoxicillin
-mab	Monoclonal antibodies	trastuzumab, abciximab canakinumab, adalimumab belimumab, alemtuzumab bezlotoxumab and basiliximab
-statin	HMG-CoA reductase inhibitors	rosuvastatin, atorvastatin, lovastatin, simvastatin and fluvastatin
-pril	ACE inhibitors	lisinopril, enalapril, captopril, ramipril, imidapril and benazepril
-olol	Beta-blockers	atenolol, propranolol, labetalol, bucindolol, timolol, sotalol, carteolol carvedilol nadolol oxprenolol, penbutolol, pindolol
-sartan	Angiotensin receptor blockers	losartan, telmisartan, valsartan

Brand names
Brand names are the names pharmaceutical companies give to drugs that have been tried, tested and approved by regulatory bodies. Brand names are also called trade names. Many drugs have multiple trade names that differ from country to country.

Examples of trade names of common generic drugs

Zoloft – sertraline
Advil – ibuprofen
Tylenol – acetaminophen
Viagra – sildenafil
Rocephin – ceftriaxone
Lipitor – atorvastatin
Benadryl – diphenhydramine
Aspirin – acetylsalicylic acid
Claritin – loratadine

Naming rules
Naming rules govern how proprietary and generic names are written.

Generic names start with a lowercase letter, while trade names start with a capital letter. Nonproprietary names are written first. The trade name is then written in parentheses. These rules are particularly important for research and science journals to prevent conflict of interest. Exceptions are applied to trade names that start with a sentence, brand names with intercapping, and nonproprietary names that use tall man letters within the drug name.

Classifications of drugs

Drugs are classified according to their similarities. Drug classification is useful in ensuring the safety of a drug during its use in the following ways:

Drug-drug interactions – When drugs are classified by their mechanisms of action, it becomes easier to identify drugs with antagonistic, agonistic, potentiating and inhibiting effects. For example, antacids that reduce the acidity of the stomach by binding to H+ can have antagonistic effects on drugs that depend on H+ for absorption (iron supplements) and protease inhibitors.

Drug clearance – The clearance of drugs also depends on their metabolism by specific liver enzymes. For example, using two drugs that are metabolized by a common liver enzyme can reduce the rate at which these drugs are metabolized. This can cause a buildup of metabolites in the liver and lead to toxicity. Furthermore, some drugs can upregulate certain liver enzymes, which can hasten the clearance of other drugs. These drugs are called inducers. Examples of inducers include carbamazepine, which hastens clearance of theophylline, and common psychiatric drugs like tricyclic antidepressants (TCAs) and antipsychotics.

Other drugs can downregulate certain liver enzymes and slow down the clearance of certain drugs. These drugs can become toxic to the liver or cause serious side or adverse effects. These drugs are called inhibitors. An example is cimetidine, which can slow down the metabolism of antidepressants and antipsychotics.

Drug resistance – Drug classification also reduces the risk of drug resistance. This is particularly important for antimicrobial drugs. Health-care providers often prescribe drugs from different classes to reduce the risk of resistance to infectious diseases.

Drugs are classified according to:

Comprehensive systems

ATC system

This is the Anatomical Chemical Classification System. It was created by the WHO in 1976. Drugs are classified according to five levels.

Level 1 (organ system) – Drugs are classified according to the system of the body receiving the therapeutic effects. There are 9 letters used in this classification system:

A – Drugs for the alimentary tract
B – Drugs for the blood and hematologic system
C – Cardiovascular drugs
D – Dermatologicals
G – Drugs for the genitourinary system and sex organs
N – Drugs for the nervous systems
M – Musculoskeletal drugs
R – Drugs for the respiratory system
S – Drugs for the sensory organs, antiparasitics, systemic anti-infectives, immunomodulating drugs, antineoplastic drugs and more

Level 2 (therapeutic action) – Drugs are classified according to a drug's therapeutic action. This classification is made up of two digits. For example, drugs classified as C by level 1 are cardiovascular drugs. Subgroups of this class include C01 – Cardiac therapy; C05 – Vasoprotectives; C07 – Beta-blockers; C09 – Drugs that act on the renin-angiotensin system, and so on.

Level 3 (mechanism of action) – Drugs are classified according to their mechanism of action. This classification is made up of a letter.

Level 4 (chemical properties) – Drugs are classified according to their pharmacological or chemical properties. This classification is made up of a letter.

Level 5 (chemical components) – Drugs are classified according to their chemical components or substances. This classification is made up of two digits.

USP drug classification

This classification was created by the United States Pharmacopeia (USP) in 1820. Drugs are classified according to their therapeutic action, mechanism of action and formulary. There are 51 classes of drugs, with numerous subclasses.

Classification according to the chemical class

Drugs are classified according to the structure of their compounds (fibrate, steroids, triptans, cardiac glycoside, B-lactam antibiotic).

Classification according to the mechanism of action

Drugs are classified according to their action on biological receptors. They can act as antagonists, agonists, inverse agonists and modulators on receptors. Examples include beta-blockers, ACE inhibitors, renin inhibitors, selective serotonin reuptake inhibitors, proton pump inhibitors, HMG-CoA reductase inhibitors, dopamine agonists, alpha-adrenergic agonists and cholinergic agonists.

Mode of action

Drugs are classified according to the form of physiologic or anatomical change they produce. Examples include antidiuretic drugs, chronotropes, antithrombotics, antifungal drugs, laxatives, decongestants, bronchodilators and diuretics.

Therapeutic class

Drugs are classified according to the pathology they treat. Examples include antibiotics, antidiabetics, antidepressants, antipsychotics, antiepileptics, antiretrovirals, cardiovascular drugs, stimulants, sedatives, anxiolytics, mood stabilizers, disease-modifying antirheumatic drugs, anticoagulants, antihypertensive drugs and antiplatelets.

Legal classification

This includes drugs classified under the pregnancy category or controlled substances.

Pregnancy category

This classification is used to assess the risk of a drug's harm to a fetus when transferred via the fetomaternal circulation. It does not cover drugs transferred through breast milk.

Categories include:

A – This includes drugs with no risks demonstrated during controlled human trials. Trials did not show risks to fetuses during the first trimester and later trimesters of pregnancy.

B – This includes drugs with no fetal risk demonstrated during animal trials, with insufficient well-controlled human trials. It also includes drugs that have demonstrated adverse fetal risks in animal trials but have not demonstrated risks to the fetus in well-controlled human trials.

C – This includes drugs whose risks have not been ruled out. In these drugs, adverse effects have been demonstrated in animal trials, but there is insufficient data on well-controlled trials in pregnant women. Drugs are used if the benefits outweigh the potential risks to the fetus.

D – This includes drugs with demonstrated risk to the human fetus. Data is obtained from well-controlled human trials and marketing or investigational research. However, the drug can be used if the benefits outweigh the risks to the fetus.

X – This category of drugs is contraindicated in pregnancy. Well-controlled human trials and animal trials have shown fetal risks, adverse reactions and fetal abnormalities. The drugs have risks that outweigh their benefits.

N – These are drugs that have not yet been classified by the FDA into a pregnancy category.

Schedules for controlled substances

In this classification, drugs are classified based on their tendency for abuse, the potential for addiction and medical use.

Schedule I – This category of drugs has a high potential for abuse and addiction. It is not safe for medical use even under the strictest professional supervision. Examples include alpha-methyltryptamine, a psychedelic drug; benzylpiperazine, a stimulant drug; heroin, an opioid; cathinone, an amphetamine derivative; dimethyltryptamine, a psychedelic drug; etorphine, a semi-synthetic opioid; gamma-hydroxybutyric acid, a sedative; mescaline; ibogaine; lysergic acid diethylamide; MDMA, psilocybin; and psilocin.

Schedule II – This category of drugs has a high potential for abuse. However, it may be used for medical conditions with strict supervision and precautions. Examples include amphetamines, cocaine, barbiturates, pure codeine, fentanyl, hydrocodone, pure diphenoxylate, hydromorphone, morphine, cannabinoids, oxycodone, oxymorphone, methylphenidate, nabilone, pethidine and phencyclidine.

Schedule III – This category of drugs has a medium risk for abuse. It is used for medical treatment, although abuse causes severe mental addiction. Examples include ketamine, anabolic steroids, dihydrocodeine, buprenorphine, marinol, xyrem, paregoric, fast-acting barbiturates, ergine, phendimetrazine, benzphetamine HCl and carbrital.

Schedule IV – This category of drugs has a moderate risk for abuse. It is used for medical treatment, although abuse causes moderate mental addiction. Examples include benzodiazepines, long-acting barbiturates, benzodiazepine-like Z-drugs, opioid partial agonists, tramadol, difenoxin and modafinil.

Schedule V – This category of drugs has a mild risk for abuse. It is used for medical treatment, although abuse causes mild mental addiction. Examples include codeine in cough syrups, anticonvulsants like retigabine, pregabalin, centrally acting antimotility drugs like diphenoxylate when mixed with atropine, and cannabidiol.

Therapeutic Equivalence

This is used to describe two drugs that have the same pharmacodynamics and pharmacokinetics and can therefore be safely substituted for the other. For two drugs to be therapeutic equivalents, they must be approved by the FDA as effective and safe for use, meet standards of quality, strength, purity and identity, and be bioequivalent. They must be properly labeled and manufactured according to the manufacturing guidelines.

Therapeutic equivalence is applicable only to drugs with the same active ingredients. It is not used to describe drugs that have different active ingredients but treat the same condition. They can, however, differ in the way they are configured, shaped, scored, packaged, released and have added excipients.

Pharmaceutical equivalents – These are two drugs that contain the same active ingredient and have the same dosage, route of administration, drug concentration and drug strength. They can, however, differ in the way they are configured, shaped, scored, packaged, released and have added excipients.

Pharmaceutical alternatives – These are drugs that have the same active ingredient expressed in different esters, salts or complexes. The term is also used to describe drugs with the same active ingredient in a different dosage, strength or form.

Bioequivalence – Drugs are bioequivalent if they have the same bioavailability at the same dose. This means that both drugs have the same pharmacokinetics.

Pharmacodynamics

This is the study of molecular, physiologic and biochemical effects of drugs on body tissues. It involves the study of chemical interactions, receptor binding and post-receptor effects. Concepts in pharmacodynamics include:

Drug effects – Drugs act by inducing physiological processes or inhibiting pathologic processes. The seven main forms of drug action are:

1. Stimulation of receptors
2. Inhibition of receptors
3. Antagonist action
4. Stabilization
5. Replacing substances or reserving them
6. Direct useful chemical reactions, like free radicals scavenging
7. Direct harmful chemical reactions, like cytotoxicity

Receptor binding – Receptors are used for chemical signaling within a cell and from one cell to the other. They are found on the surface of the cell membrane or in the cytoplasm of the cell. When receptors are activated, they regulate cellular functions either directly or indirectly. Some of these cellular functions include enzymatic activity, protein phosphorylation, ion conductance and DNA transcription.

Molecules like hormones, drugs and neurotransmitters bind to receptors. They are called ligands. Such infections can be reversible or irreversible. This binding can activate or inactivate a receptor and consequently inhibit or stimulate a cellular function(s).

Drugs demonstrate:

Selectivity – The extent to which a drug acts on a site with other sites.

Affinity – The probability of a drug occupying a receptor. The affinity of a drug to a receptor can be affected by both intracellular and external factors. Factors like aging, genetic disorders and mutations can increase or decrease the affinity of receptors.

Intrinsic efficacy – The extent to which a drug will activate a receptor antagonist

Residence time – This is the time spent by a drug-receptor complex. It is affected by changes to the conformation of the receptor that controls how long the drug will act on or dissociate from the receptor.

Agonists – Agonists bind to receptors and activate them to stimulate a desired cellular response. Conventional agonists increase the number of activated receptors. Inverse agonists, on the other hand, make the inactive receptor stable and therefore stimulate responses similar to competitive antagonists.

Antagonists – Antagonists bind to receptors and prevent their activation to block certain cellular functions or increase certain functions that are blocked by certain cellular substrates. By binding to these substrates, antagonists can increase cellular functions.

Reversible antagonists dissociate from receptors, while irreversible antagonists do not. Irreversible antagonists form a stable or permanent bond with the receptor.

Competitive antagonism – The agonist and antagonist compete for the same receptor. When the antagonist binds to the receptor, the agonist is unable to bind.

Noncompetitive antagonism – Both the agonist and antagonist bind to the receptor, but the antagonist reduces the action of the agonist on the receptor.

Reversible competitive antagonism – Both the antagonist and agonist temporarily bind to the receptor. The effects of the antagonist can be overcome if the concentration of the agonist is increased.

Partial agonists – These agonists have both agonist and antagonistic properties. They act as agonists when they are the only molecules bound to the receptors. However, when another agonist binds to the receptor, it becomes antagonistic. For example, pentazocine has agonistic effects on opioid receptors but becomes antagonistic if another opioid binds to the receptor.

Pharmacokinetics

This is the study of how drugs are absorbed, distributed, metabolized and excreted.

Drug absorption

Factors that affect the rate of absorption are the drug's formulation, physicochemical properties and route of administration. However, regardless of the formulation of a drug, it must be dissolved in a solution for it to be absorbed.

For drugs to reach the circulation, they must cross through cell membranes by using any of these methods:

Passive diffusion – The drugs pass through the cell membrane across a gradient (from an area of high concentration in the gut to an area of low concentration in the blood). The rate of passive diffusion is proportional to the gradient of the concentration. It is also affected by the solubility of the lipid molecules of the drug, the size of the molecules, the surface area of the membrane and the level of ionization of the molecule.

Molecules that are lipid soluble diffuse the fastest. Small molecules diffuse faster than large ones. Un-ionized molecules are typically soluble in lipids and thus diffuse faster than ionized ones. The amount of a drug's un-ionized molecules is determined by both the drug's pKa and the environment's pH. If pKa is higher than the pH, the molecules are predominantly in un-ionized forms of the weak acids and ionized forms of the weak base.

Facilitated passive diffusion – The molecules are transported across the cell membrane by a carrier molecule. For example, glucose has low solubility in lipids. It is quickly diffused by carrier molecules (glucose transporters). These carrier molecules bind to glucose, pass the membrane barrier and quickly dissociate from glucose. This movement does not need energy. ATP and transport are down a concentration gradient.

Active transport – This form of cellular transport requires an expenditure of energy. Transport can occur upward on a concentration gradient. This form of transport is useful for drugs in the form of endogenous substrates (vitamins), ions, amino acids and sugars.

Pinocytosis – The molecules are engulfed by cells. The engulfed molecules are transported into the cytoplasm in the form of a vesicle. This transport method requires energy expenditure.

Oral administration of drugs

Absorption of oral drugs is affected by gut pH, surface area, mucus, bile, blood perfusion and the nature of the epithelia. The epithelia in the oral mucosa are thin. This makes oral mucosa ideal for absorption of sublingual drugs or drugs placed between the cheek and gums.

Although the stomach has a large surface area, it has a thick mucosa and a short transit time that can affect the rate of drug absorption. For these reasons, drug absorption occurs primarily in the small intestine. The rate of absorption in the small intestine is affected by the rate of gastric emptying. Food—particularly food rich in fat—delays gastric emptying time. The transit time of the intestine can affect the rate of absorption. This is particularly true for drugs that require active transportation, drugs with low solubility in lipids and drugs that dissolve slowly.

Parenteral administration

Drugs that are given intravenously enter the systemic circulation immediately. Drugs that are given intramuscularly or subcutaneously cross a few cell membrane barriers before entering the systemic circulation. Drugs that are coupled to proteins with large molecular weight are slow to cross the capillary membranes. Circulation is almost always through the lymphatic system. Perfusion affects the rate of absorption of other parenteral routes apart from IV.

Drug distribution

Drugs are distributed into tissues via systemic circulation. The rate and extent of distribution are determined by tissue binding, the extent of perfusion, permeability of membranes, regional pH, the type of partition between tissue and blood and tissue mass.

Volume of distribution

Apparent volume of distribution – This is the amount of fluid that should contain the drug to reach plasma concentration. It is a theoretical value because it does not factor in the actual amount of fluid in the body's compartments. It is strictly focused on how the drug is distributed in the body. Drugs that stay in circulation have low volumes of distribution. Although the volume of distribution gives rough estimates on plasma concentration, it does not say much about the pattern of distribution.

For example, some drugs are distributed in adipose tissues, while some are distributed to the extracellular fluid or bind to specific tissues. Acidic drugs have small volumes of distribution because they are bound to protein. Basic drugs, on the other hand, can have large volumes of distribution because they are used up by tissues.

Binding

The distribution of drugs depends on binding to plasma proteins or tissues. In the systemic circulation, drugs are transported as unbound drugs, drugs that are partially bound to plasma proteins. While acidic drugs are mostly bound to albumin, basic drugs bind readily to lipoproteins and alpha-1-acid glycoprotein. The unbound molecules readily pass through the cell membrane via passive diffusion. This means that the efficacy of a drug is determined by the unbound molecules.

If drug concentrations are very high, the quantity of bound molecules reaches an upper limit. Saturation sets in, and a displacement reaction occurs. Apart from carrier proteins, drugs can also bind to fat cells. This can reduce the rate of metabolism and excretion of the drug because fat cells have poor perfusion.

Drugs that accumulate in body tissues and compartments for a long time have a longer duration of action.

Blood-brain barrier (BBB)

Drugs enter the central nervous system (CNS) through the cerebrospinal fluid (CSF). Drugs enter the CSF through capillaries in the brain. However, the permeability of drugs to the brain is restricted via the blood-brain barrier. This barrier is made of tightly packed endothelial cells covered by an astrocytic sheath. The endothelial cells are impermeable to water-soluble molecules. However, drugs can enter the CSF through the choroid plexus then diffuse passively from the CSF. The absorption of drugs via the BBB is determined by the degree of ionization, protein binding and the lipid-to-water partition coefficient of the molecule.

Drug metabolism

Drugs are metabolized primarily in the liver into inactive metabolites. However, in rare cases, metabolites of some drugs are more active than the parent molecule. Drugs with this kind of characteristic are called prodrugs. Metabolic processes include oxidation, hydrolysis, reduction, isomerization, condensation and conjugation.

Rate of metabolism

The rate of metabolism is affected by genetics, medical disorders that affect the liver and drug interactions that can inhibit or induce certain liver enzymes. The rate of metabolism can be first-order kinetics, meaning that the rate of metabolism is in proportion to the fraction of drugs left. It can also be in zero-order kinetics, meaning that the rate of metabolism is maximum, and a fixed amount of drug is metabolized per time. As the concentration of a drug increases, the metabolic rate typically switches from first order to zero order.

Enzymes

The enzymes involved in phase I metabolism are the cytochrome P-450 (CYP450) enzymes. These enzymes are involved in oxidation. These enzymes can be inhibited or induced by drugs and substrates that can trigger drug interactions that can either reduce the therapeutic effect of the drug or increase its toxicity.

Conjugation

The most common form of phase II reaction is glucuronidation. It occurs in the liver microsomes. After this, the glucuronides are conjugated and then secreted into the bile. They are finally excreted in the urine. The purpose of conjugation is to make drug metabolites soluble so that they can be excreted by the kidneys. Other forms of conjugation include sulfoconjugation and acetylation.

Renal excretion

Drug metabolites are excreted primarily via the kidneys because they are water-soluble and have a higher polarity. Renal excretion of drugs decreases as one ages. Another factor that affects renal excretion is the pH of the urine. Acidic urine reduces the rate at which weak acids are excreted. It also stimulates reabsorption. Alkalinizing the urine improves the rate of excretion of weak acids. Furthermore, metabolic inhibitors can slow down the rate of excretion in the proximal tubule of the nephron.

Hepatic excretion

Excretion in the bile is done via active transport because excretion is down against a gradient. Metabolites excreted in the bile are eliminated through the feces.

Common and Life-Threatening Drug Interactions and Contraindications

Drug-drug

Drug-drug interactions can occur on the level of pharmacokinetics and pharmacodynamics.

Pharmacodynamic drug interactions
These are interactions that occur at the level of the drug's receptor. Common pharmacodynamic interactions include:

Myocardial infarction – Patients who are on acetylsalicylic acid (ASA) for coronary artery disease should avoid taking ibuprofen because it binds reversibly to COX-1 and prevents the irreversible binding of ASA to COX-1 receptors. Because ASA is unable to bind to COX-1, it is unable to acetylate the serine molecule on the COX-1 protein. This failure stimulates the synthesis of thromboxane A2, a mediator that stimulates platelet aggregation and increases the risk of myocardial infarction in patients with coronary artery disease.

Hyperkalemia – ACE inhibitors (ACEIs) like captopril should not be used with potassium-sparing diuretics like amiloride. Their drug interaction can increase the risk of hyperkalemia, which is often life-threatening.

Gastrointestinal bleeding – NSAIDs should not be taken together with selective serotonin reuptake inhibitors (SSRIs) like citalopram because their pharmacodynamic interactions increase the risk of gastrointestinal bleeding. NSAIDs bind to COX-1 and prevent platelet aggregation. SSRIs, on the other hand, block the transport of serotonin into platelets and thereby prevent platelet aggregation. These combined effects increase the risk of gastrointestinal bleeding. SSRIs should not also be taken together with vitamin K antagonists like warfarin because of the increased risk of bleeding.

Blood pressure – NSAIDs can inhibit the blood pressure–lowering effect of ACEIs. Since NSAIDs block prostaglandin synthesis and reduce perfusion in the glomerulus, they can trigger a reactive renin secretion, which can inhibit the action of ACEIs.

Serotonin syndrome – Concomitant use of SSRIs and triptans can trigger serotonin syndrome.

Torsade de Pointes – Concomitant use of quinolones and macrolides or quinolones and citalopram can trigger Torsade de Pointes.

Pharmacokinetic drug interactions

Level of absorption

Calcium supplements and antacids containing calcium carbonate can inhibit the absorption of bisphosphonates, levothyroxine, quinolones and tetracycline. They do so by forming complexes with them.

Membrane transport

Drugs can increase or decrease the availability of other drugs by inducing or inhibiting efflux transporters like P-glycoprotein.

Inhibitors and inducers of P-glycoprotein

Substrates	Inducers	Inhibitors
Ciclosporin	Carbamazepine	Ciclosporin
Digoxin	Rifampicin	Verapamil
Aliskiren	Primidone	Amiodarone
Dabigatran	Efavirenz	Erythromycin
Indinavir	St. John's wort extract	Indinavir
Paclitaxel	Phenytoin	Itraconazole
Loperamide	Hyperforin	
Atorvastatin	Phenobarbital	

At the level of metabolism

This happens when cytochrome P450 enzymes (CYP) in the liver lysosomes are either inhibited or induced. Common interactions include:

Anticoagulants – Interactions of old-generation macrolide antibiotics, like clarithromycin and erythromycin, can inhibit cytochrome P450 3A4 and inhibit the metabolism of warfarin. Other inhibitors that should not be used with anticoagulants include verapamil (a calcium channel blocker), ketoconazole and fluconazole.

Antidepressants – SSRIs inhibit CYP2D6 and CYP1A2. These drugs can increase the bioavailability of some beta-blockers, clozapine and theophylline.

Quinolones – Quinolones, like ciprofloxacin and ofloxacin, inhibit CYP1A2 and can increase the bioavailability of theophylline.

Proton pump inhibitors (PPIs) – PPIs inhibit CYP2C19. This inhibits the conversion of the prodrug clopidogrel into its active metabolite. Concomitant use increases the risk of acute coronary syndrome in patients with coronary artery disease. PPIs increase the bioavailability of citalopram and increase the risk of QT prolongation. They also increase the bioavailability of diazepam.

Drug-dietary supplement interaction

Complementary drugs	Interacting drug	Outcome
Calcium supplements	Thyroxine, quinolone antibiotics and tetracycline	Decreased drug action
Black cohosh	Cisplatin	Decreased action of cisplatin
Gingko	Anticonvulsant	Increased risk for seizures
Ginger	Warfarin and antiplatelet drugs	Increased risk for bleeding
Ginseng	Warfarin and antiplatelet drugs	Increased for bleeding
Hawthorn	Antidiabetic drugs	Hyperglycemia
Kava	Calcium channel blockers	Increased drug effect

Drug-nutrient interactions

Citrus – Citrus fruits contain naringin, a flavonoid that inhibits CYP3A4 and increases the bioavailability of midazolam and anticoagulants.

Milk – The calcium in milk binds to quinolones, bisphosphonates and tetracyclines and prevents their absorption.

Aged and fermented foods – Aged cheeses, cured meats, red wine, pickled vegetables, fermented soy and others contain tyramine, a neurotransmitter.

When eaten in significant amounts, it can interact with MAOIs and trigger a hypertensive crisis.

Grapefruit – Grapefruits inhibit CYP3A4 and can increase the bioavailability of a good number of drugs to toxic levels. Some of the drugs affected by grapefruit include midazolam, felodipine, cyclosporine, most psychotropics, anticonvulsants and anticoagulants.

Vegetables – Vegetables that are high in vitamin K (kale), Brussel sprouts, spinach and parsley can inhibit the action of warfarin.

Cranberry juice – Cranberries can induce or inhibit a significant amount of cytochrome p450 enzymes and affect the bioavailability of drugs. Cranberries can inhibit the metabolism of warfarin.

Licorice – Licorice contains glycyrrhizin, which can inhibit 11-beta-hydroxysteroid dehydrogenase and induce potassium secretion and retention of sodium. It can interfere with both antiarrhythmics and antihypertensives.

Alcohol – Alcohol should not be taken with NSAIDs, as it increases the risk of gastrointestinal bleeding and liver damage. Alcohol should not be taken with metronidazole, as it induces a disulfiram-like effect. Alcohol can increase the risk of irritability and nausea if taken with theophylline. Generally, alcohol should not be taken with drugs.

Drug-laboratory interaction

1. Cephalosporins can create false-positive glucose results in the urine.
2. Ranitidine and labetalol can create false-positive results for amphetamines.
3. Rifampin can create false-positive results for opioids.
4. Telavancin and daptomycin can create false-positive results for elevated prothrombin time and INR.
5. Acetaminophen, albuterol, lisinopril and atenolol can cause false-positive results of serum hyperglycemia.

Drug-disease interactions

This is a concern for older adults who are at risk for polypharmacy for multiple disorders.

1. Antipsychotics can cause symptoms that mimic Parkinson's disease.
2. Cholinesterase inhibitors used to treat dementia can cause urge incontinence, diarrhea and urinary frequency.
3. Calcium channel blockers used for treating hypertension can cause peripheral edema.
4. Patients with chronic renal disease can suffer from worsening renal function if given NSAIDs, gentamicin, amphotericin B and other nephrotoxic drugs.
5. Patients with tinnitus, deafness or other auditory problems should not be given thiazides, aminoglycosides and certain antimalarials.
6. Patients with Crohn's disease, celiac disease and other forms of inflammatory bowel disease should not be given NSAIDs.

Strength/Dose

Dose – This is the amount of drug administered at a particular time.

Dosage – This includes the number of doses of a medication administered over a period, including the frequency of administration and the number of drugs.

Concentration – This is the number of active ingredients per total weight of a medication.

Alligation – This is a process of combining solids or solutions with various strengths to get another strength of the active ingredients.

Specific gravity – This is the proportion of a substance's weight to that of an equal volume of water.

Isotonicity – When two different solutions have the same osmotic pressure and concentration of salt, they demonstrate isotonicity. Normal saline is an isotonic crystalloid because it has the same osmotic pressure as the plasma.

Percent strength – This is the number of grams dissolved in 100 mL of a solution.

Percent weight in volume (w/v) – This is the number of grams in 100 mL of a solution. It is used to measure solid substances like powders.

Percent volume in volume (v/v) – This is the number of milliliters in 100 mL of a solution in % v/v. It is used to measure liquid substances mixed with a liquid preparation.

Percent weight in weight (w/w) – This is the number of grams in 100 g of a solution. It is measured in % w/w. It is used to measure powdered substances prepared with semisolid or solid substances.

The following calculations are useful in measuring drug dosages:

Number of tablets = desired dose/stick strength

Amount of solution to be administered = [desired dose/stock strength] × stock volume

IV Rate (mL per hour and minute) = Total IV Volume/Time (hour or minute)

Drops per minute = [Total IV volume/Time (minute)] X Drop Factor

Remaining time of infusion = [Volume remaining (in mL)/Drops per minute] x Drop Factor

Dosage Forms

Solid drugs

Tablets – Tablets are made by compressing drug powders and then bulking them up with fillers. The route of administration of tablets depends on their form. For example, some tablets should be swallowed whole with water, some should be inserted as suppositories, and some should be dissolved in the mouth. Subtypes of tablets include enteric-coated tablets, sublingual tablets, chewable tablets, buccal tablets and buffered tablets.

Chewable tablets must be crushed before they are swallowed. They often have a sugar base or are flavored to improve palatability (antacids). Sublingual tablets are placed underneath the tongue for rapid absorption (nitroglycerin). Buccal tablets are placed between the gum and the cheek for rapid absorption. Enteric-coated tablets are coated to prevent erosion by gastric acid in the stomach. This allows the drug to pass through the stomach and be dissolved in the intestine. Buffered tablets are prepared with antacids to prevent them from ulcerating the gastric mucosa.

Pills – Pills are single doses of a drug made by adding a syrup into a powdered drug and then rolling the mixture into an oval or round shape.

Plasters – Plasters are a mixture of powder and liquid that becomes hard when dry. Plasters can be semisolid or solid (salicylic acid plaster used to treat corns).
Capsules – In this drug form, the medication is contained in a gelatinous shell. Gelatin shells are used to enclose granules, liquids, powders or a combination of these. They are ideally used for drugs with unpleasant tastes or odors. Sustained-release capsules should never be dissolved or crushed because doing so can affect their timed release.

Caplets – Caplets are shaped like capsules but are in the form of tablets. They are designed this way to make them easier to swallow.

Gel caps – Gel caps are oil based and covered by a gelatinous shell.

Powders – Powder is ground into fine particles (most antifungal drugs for the foot, potassium chloride powder and nystatin powder).

Granules – Granules are small and numerous and enclosed by a gelatinous shell. They are designed for slow release.

Troches – Also called lozenges, troches are flattened semisolid or hard drugs. Troches are placed in the sublingual or buccal mucosa for absorption (clotrimazole). An example is cetylpyridinium chloride.

Semisolid drugs

These drugs are applied topically because they are pliable and soft. Examples include ointments, suppositories, pessaries, gels, lotions and pastes.

Suppositories – Suppositories are shaped like bullets and inserted into an orifice (for example, the rectum). The drug acts locally at the site of insertion. It dissolves when inserted but is solid at room temperature.

Ointments – Ointments are made with oil to form a semisolid consistency. They are applied topically (anesthetics, antibiotics and anti-inflammatory drugs).

Creams – Creams are semisolid, non-greasy dose forms. They are typically colored white and applied to the skin or mucosa (vagina).

Gels – Gels are jelly-like and are applied topically. Some gels have a high amount of alcohol and can sting broken skin.

Lotions – Lotions are semisolid and are applied topically to protect the skin or treat skin disorders.

Pastes – Pastes are semisolid drug formulations. They have a fatty base (zinc oxide paste).

Patches – These are adhesive patches that are applied to the skin. The drug is absorbed by the skin and sent into the systemic circulation (nitroglycerin, scopolamine, nicotine, antidepressants, contraceptives and others).

All of the above are discussed in more detail later in the book.

Liquid drugs

Syrups – Syrups contain a high amount of sucrose (ipecac syrup).

Solutions – Solutions have a drug powder dissolved in them.

Spirits – Spirits have alcohol as a solvent. They are also called essences (essence of peppermint).

Elixirs – Elixirs are made up of sugar, water and alcohol. They may be aromatic and may or may not be medicinal. Since all elixirs contain alcohol, they should be cautiously used in patients with diabetes or alcohol addiction.

Tinctures – Tinctures are a drug form in which alcohol is the primary solvent (iodine tincture).

Fluid extracts – Fluid extracts are liquid concentrates sourced from a plant. After the plant is dissolved in alcohol, the residue is filtered out. Fluid extracts are not given to patients directly. They are used to manufacture drugs.

Liniments – Liniments are made by mixing drugs with soap, water, oil or alcohol. The mixture is used topically (chloroform liniment).

Emulsions – Emulsions are made by mixing two substances that ordinarily do not mix well together (dispersing oil in water).

Mixtures/suspensions – Mixtures or suspensions are mixed with a liquid but do not dissolve into the liquid (milk of magnesia).

Aromatic water – This is made by mixing distilled water into an aromatic oil.

Sprays/aerosols – These are made by mixing powder or liquid into a mist. They are typically used for respiratory treatments.

Many of the above are discussed more in detail later in the book.

Gaseous drugs

Gaseous drugs are commonly used for anesthesia (halothane and nitrous oxide) and compressed gases like carbon dioxide and oxygen.

Routes of administration

The route of drug administration affects the rate at which a drug is absorbed. It also affects the intensity of the drug's actions. The routes of administration include:

Oral route

This is the safest way to administer drugs. It is also very convenient. It includes all drugs taken by mouth. Basic materials used for administering oral drugs include medicine cups, water cups, droppers, spoons and oral syringes.

Parenteral route

This includes administering drugs that bypass the digestive system. It includes drugs administered through the veins, muscles, skin or spinal column.

Materials needed for parenteral administration include disposable needles, nondisposable needles and all sorts of medication containers (sterile cartridges, vials and ampoules).

Ampoules have scoured weak points on their necks, while vials have rubber stoppers through which needles are inserted. Vials can be single dose or multiple dose. While single-dose vials are used for a single administration, multiple-dose vials are used more than once. Multiple-dose vials have a high risk for contamination. Care should be taken when withdrawing doses from these vials to prevent contamination.

Forms of parenteral medication

Parenteral drugs are formulated as powders or solutions. Powders are not injected but are dissolved with a liquid before they are used. Solutions, on the other hand, are injected directly. They must be homogenous.

Intradermal injection
The common site for intradermal injection is the middle of the forearm. Other sites are the back and the upper part of the chest. The intradermal route is often used for allergy testing and tuberculin testing. The needle is angled at 15°.

Subcutaneous injection
This injection is given into the subcutaneous layer that is below the dermis and adipose tissue. The most common sites for administration are the anterior thigh, upper back, abdomen and deltoid area. The angle of insertion is 45° for allergy medications, epinephrine and local anesthetics and 90° for heparin and insulin. The maximum volume of drugs to be administered via this route is 2 mL.

IM injection
This route is suitable for vesicant drugs, drugs with large volumes and drugs that need rapid absorption. The most common sites for injection are the deltoid, vastus lateralis and gluteus maximus. The vastus lateralis, which is located in the anterolateral surface of the thigh, is the safest site for infants. It is part of the quadriceps muscle. The angle of insertion is 90°.

The deltoid muscle is not an acceptable injection site for infants but is safe enough for older children. Adults can tolerate about 2 mL of a drug into the deltoid muscle and 5 mL in the gluteus and vastus lateralis. Infants should not be given more than 2 mL in the vastus lateralis and gluteus.

IV injection
This route is suitable for emergencies because of the rapid onset of drugs administered via this route. The most commonly used veins in adults are the dorsal, metacarpal, cephalic and basilic veins. In infants, veins on the dorsum of the foot and scalp can be used.

Pump systems
This route is used to continuously administer drugs to patients. Pumps are electrical devices used to pump a specific amount of IV solution through a patient's vein at a preset time. For example, pump systems are used to administer insulin to diabetics and opioids to terminally ill patients.

Urethral route
In this route, a solution is pumped into the bladder via a urethral catheter.

Topical route
In this route, medications are applied to the skin or mucosa for their local effects (buccal, rectal, subcutaneous and vaginal topical applications). Another form of a topical route is a transdermal patch, which is applied to the skin for sustained and controlled release. The drug is absorbed by the capillaries of the skin and sent into the systemic circulation.

Inhalational route
This includes gases, vapors and medicines suspended in water vapor. Drugs administered via this route have a local effect on the respiratory system.

Ophthalmic route
This includes eye drops and eye ointments. Ophthalmic drugs must be sterile, and the process of applying them must also be sterile to avoid conjunctivitis. Drugs administered via this route include antivirals, antibiotics, topical anesthetics, artificial tears and decongestants.

Otic route
This route is used for treating ear infections. It is contraindicated for perforated eardrums. When applying ear drops for children (less than three years), the earlobe should be pulled down and back. For adults and older children, it should be pulled upward and outward. After application, the patient should be advised to stay on the same side for at least five minutes to allow gravity to work.

Nasal route
This route is used to treat nasal infections or congestions. Drugs should be applied one nostril at a time. Note that nasal medications are often abused by patients.

Vaginal route
This route includes tablets, suppositories, creams and liquids. These drugs are effective when the patient lies down.

Rectal route

This route is suitable for unconscious, nauseated or vomiting patients. Rectal drugs are often made with gelatin or cocoa butter. They are solid at room temperature and melt when inserted. Rectal suppositories should be administered after an enema or bowel movement.

Common and Severe Medication Side Effects, Adverse Effects and Allergies

Side effects

These are secondary effects caused by a drug. They can be therapeutic or adverse. Although side effects describe unwanted, unpleasant effects, they also include unexpected beneficial effects.

Examples of therapeutic side effects include:

1. Bupropion, an antidepressant used to help patients with nicotine dependence
2. Carbamazepine, an antiseizure drug used to treat patients with post-traumatic stress disorder, phantom limb syndrome, attention-deficit hyperactivity disorder (ADHD), phantom limb pain and neuromyotonia
3. Dexamethasone, a corticosteroid used to stimulate fetal lung maturity
4. Hydroxyzine, a histamine receptor blocker used as an anxiolytic
5. Magnesium sulfate, which is used to treat preeclampsia and premature labor
6. Methotrexate, which is used to treat choriocarcinoma
7. Sildenafil, which was originally designed for pulmonary hypertension, is used to treat erectile dysfunction
8. Terazosin, which is an alpha 1 adrenergic receptor blocker used to treat benign prostatic hyperplasia, is also used to treat hyperhidrosis and diaphoresis.

Adverse effects

These are unwanted and undesirable side effects of a drug. They do not include effects caused by the inappropriate dosage or route of administration. Most adverse effects are mild and nonfatal. The most common include dizziness, nausea, diarrhea, vomiting, headache, dry mouth, dermatitis and malaise. However, adverse effects differ from person to person. Some examples of specific adverse effects include:

Misoprostol – Abortions, uterine hemorrhages and miscarriages
Opioids, sedatives, anxiolytics – Addiction, physical and mental dependence
NSAIDs and aspirin – Hypertension, gastrointestinal bleeding and liver disease
Atypical antipsychotics – Diabetes
Interferon – Depression and hepatic injury
Chemotherapy agents – Anemia, hair loss and dermatitis
Aminoglycosides – Nephrotoxicity and ototoxicity
Antidepressants – Weight gain, loss of libido, erectile dysfunction and increased risk of suicide (particularly for SSRIs)
Corticosteroids – Diabetes, Cushing syndrome, stunting and hypertension
Metformin – Lactic acidosis
Sildenafil – Postural hypotension and priapism
Antipsychotics – Tardive dyskinesia

Drug allergies

This is an abnormal reaction of the immune system to drugs. It can be immediate onset or delayed onset. Immediate onset is triggered by IgE antibodies. Delayed onset is triggered by the formation of immune complexes.

Commonly implicated drugs include antibiotics that contain penicillin. They can also include tetracyclines, NSAIDs, aspirin, chemotherapy agents, sulfa drugs, insulin, HIV drugs, monoclonal antibodies, muscle relaxants and antiseizure drugs.

Features of drug allergies include hives, itchy skin, rashes, running nose, diarrhea, swelling of the mouth and eyes. Severe reactions include angioedema characterized by swelling of the respiratory mucosa and difficulty breathing. Other severe reactions include fainting spells, hypotension and blistered skin.

Indications of medications and dietary supplements

Indication means that a drug is used for treating a specific condition. Drugs can have more than one indication for use.

Indications can be:

Labeled – This is also called FDA-approved indication. The indications of the drugs have been tested and verified by FDA-approved clinical trials. FDA-approved drugs are authorized to label their indications. This information can be used for marketing. Drug manufacturers are not authorized to market their drugs for indications that are not approved by the FDA.

Off-label – These are indications that have not been approved by the FDA. It is common for a drug to have therapeutic side effects. These side effects can make physicians prescribe or use these drugs to treat certain conditions. Off-label indications can have research studies that support their uses, but these studies are not as extensive as those of labeled indications.

Drug manufacturers can decide not to apply for FDA approval for certain reasons. One reason is that the number of patients in need of the drug is small, and sales of the drugs are unlikely to generate enough revenue to offset the cost of extensive studies needed by the FDA. Another reason is the presence of a similar FDA-approved drug on the market. Furthermore, there can be a lot of similar off-label alternatives in the market that can make the process of getting FDA approval seem unnecessary. Labeled and off-label indications are more important to the manufacturer than to the patient because most drug references are made up of labeled indications.

Drug Stability

Drug stability is the ability of a drug to retain its strength, identity, purity and quality. Unstable drugs can lose the efficacy of their active ingredients, vehicle, bioavailability and uniformity. They can also contain toxic metabolites.

Factors affecting the stability of a drug include microbial contamination, environmental factors and drug containers.

Environmental factors

This includes light, temperature and moisture.

Temperature – Drugs should be stored at ideal temperatures. Drugs stored at room temperature are stored from 25°C to 30°C. Drugs stored at cold temperatures are stored from 2°C to 8°C. Drugs in freeze storage are stored from -20°C to -10°C. High temperatures trigger oxidation, hydrolysis and reduction.

Light – Light rays with shorter wavelengths are readily absorbed by a drug. Degradation by light is called photolysis. To prevent photolysis, the drugs should be stored in amber-colored bottles, in aluminum foil wrappers and away from direct sunlight.

Moisture – Drugs are stored in glass or plastic containers to prevent degradation from moisture via hydrolysis.

The effect of packaging material on drug stability

Glass – Glass is durable and resistant to physical and chemical change. This property makes it a common packaging material. However, it has an alkaline surface (this challenge is overcome by using borosilicate glass). It can trigger precipitation of crystals (this can be overcome by using buffers), and it allows radiation of light rays, which can trigger degradation of light-sensitive drugs (this is overcome by tinting the glass with amber).

Plastics – Although plastics are durable like glass, they can allow the drug to migrate into the environment. They are also permeable to environmental factors like heat, oxygen and moisture. The contents of the plastic can also leach into the drug, and the active ingredients can be absorbed by the plastic.

Metals – Alloys and aluminum can be used to store ointments, pastes, creams and emulsions. They can, however, precipitate or corrode the drug. To overcome these challenges, the interior part of the containers should be coated with polymers.

Rubber – Rubber containers can leach into the drug. This challenge can be overcome by treating rubber stoppers with water or steam.

Types of degradation

Chemical degradation

Hydrolysis – The drug molecules are split by water molecules. Common drugs affected include:

1. Esters – Nitroglycerin, aspirin, dexamethasone, alkaloids
2. Lactones – Spironolactone, pilocarpine
3. Amides – Chloramphenicol
4. Malonic ureas – Barbiturates
5. Imides – Glutethimide

Oxidation – This process is characterized by a loss of hydrogen ions and electrons. Some drugs readily affected by oxidation include:

1. Ethers – Diethyl ether
2. Thioethers – Chlorpromazine
3. Carboxylic acids – Fatty acids
4. Thiols – Dimercaprol (BAL)
5. Catechols – Catecholamines

Photolysis – A good example of a drug that is affected by photolysis is sodium nitroprusside. It has a shelf life of four hours if exposed to light.

Physical degradation

A drug that undergoes physical degradation has changes in physical properties like appearance, particle size, brittleness, hardness and organoleptic properties. These changes affect the uniformity of the drug, the elegance of the drug, the drug content and the rate of release.

Examples of physical degradation include:

Formation of crystals – Caused by polyphormism

Loss of volatile gases – Can affect elixirs, nitroglycerin, aromatic water and spirits

Loss of water – Can occur in emulsions, saturated solutions, creams, pastes and ointments

Absorption – Can occur in powders that liquefy, while suppositories become jelly-like

Oral solutions – Can lose flavor, have an altered taste, discolor, precipitate and lose color. All these reactions can change the smell, taste and feel of the drug.

Emulsions – Can undergo creaming, which makes medications lose uniformity. They can also coalesce, which makes them lose elegance.

Suspensions – Can settle, cake or develop crystals. All these cause medications to lose uniformity and elegance.

Parenteral drugs – Photochemical reactions can cause discoloration. These drugs can also precipitate or become cloudy. All these changes affect the appearance and bioavailability of the drug.

Semisolids – Semisolids, like suppositories and ointments, can change in consistency and particle size. They can bleed, cake or coalesce. All these changes can affect the bioavailability, uniformity or elegance of the drug.

Tablets – Tablets can disintegrate, dissolve, become very soft and shiny or become hard. All these affect the rate of drug release.

Capsules – Capsules can change their strengths, appearances or dissolutions.

Microbial instability

Some common sources of microbial contamination include:

1. Water – Mostly gram-negative cocci (pseudomonas, flavobacterium and xanthomonas)
2. Raw materials – Micrococci
3. Pigments – Salmonella
4. Starches – Coliforms
5. Personnel – Streptococcus, staphylococcus, coliform
6. Animal products – Coliform, salmonella

How to prevent microbial contamination of formulations

1. Drug formulations should be stored in appropriate containers.
2. Drugs should also be stored in single-dose containers
3. Drugs should be stored in the appropriate storage conditions.
4. Antimicrobial agents should be used as preservatives. Examples include phenol, chlorocresol and cresol used for parenteral formulations; methylparaben used for tablets; chlorhexidine acetate used for eye drops; benzoic acid; alcohol used for mixtures; parabens; and cresol used for creams.

Factors that affect the rate of degradation

pH – The pH of a solution can influence the rate of degradation of its compound. For example, a buffered aspirin solution is stable at a pH of 2.4. If the pH increases by about 10, it quickly decomposes. The pH of a solution also influences its rate of oxidation. Solutions with low pH are not oxidized easily.

Complexation – Solutions with complexes have a lower rate of oxidation and hydrolysis. For example, caffeine is used to form a complex with procaine to reduce the rate of hydrolysis.

Surfactants – Drugs with surfactants are not easily hydrolyzed because they form a micelle and trap drug compounds inside them.

Heavy metals – Heavy metals—like iron, copper, nickel and cobalt—increase the rate of oxidation because they trigger the formation of free radicals.

Light – Light stimulates photolysis and triggers decomposition.

How to stabilize drugs against hydrolysis, photolysis and oxidation

Temperature – Drugs should be stored at the appropriate temperature to reduce the rate of decomposition.

Light – Photosensitive drugs should be stored in amber-colored bottles.

Humidity – Glass and plastic should be used to package drugs and protect them from humidity.

Antioxidants – Antioxidants are added to aqueous solutions to reduce the rate of decomposition. Common antioxidants include sodium metabisulfite used for ascorbyl palmitate, ascorbic acid used for butylated hydroxyanisole and sodium thiosulfate used for butylated hydroxytoluene.

Chelating agents – These agents form complexes with heavy metals and reduce the rate of oxidation. Commonly used chelating agents are ethylenediaminetetraacetic acid (EDTA) derivatives, tartaric acid and citric acid.

Solvents – Solvents are added to reduce the rate of hydrolysis.

Shelf life of a drug

This is the time taken for a drug to degrade to 90% of the initial strength if it is stored in ideal conditions.

Order of reaction

Zero-order reaction

Here the rate of the reaction is constant and does not depend on the concentration of the reactants.

Formula

$C - C_o = -kt$
C = concentration to be calculated
CO = initial concentration
-k = constant
t = time in years

Half-life $t_{1/2} = C_o/2k$
Shelf life = $t_{0.9} = 0.1C_o/k$

First-order reaction
This is the most common reaction. Here the rate of change depends on the concentration of the drug.

Formula

$\log c = \log c_o - kt/2.303$

Half-life $t_{1/2} = 0.693/k$
Shelf life $t_{0.9} = 0.105/k$

Second-order reaction

Here the rate of the reaction depends on the product of the two concentrations.

Formula

$1/c = 1/c_o + kt$

Half-life = $1/kC_o$
Shelf life = $0.11/kC_o$

Narrow Therapeutic Index (NTI) Medications

Therapeutic index

This is the measurement of the safety of a drug. It is also called the therapeutic ratio. It is the ratio of a drug at its therapeutic dose in 50% of subjects to its toxic dose in 50% of subjects.

Therapeutic index = TD_{50}/ED_{50}

Wide therapeutic index – Drugs with a wide therapeutic index have a wide range between the toxic dose and the effective dose. These drugs have a wide safety profile because the dose range for their therapeutic effects and lethal effects are wide apart. For toxicity to occur, very high doses are required. For example, antibiotics like B-lactams, quinolones and macrolides have a wide therapeutic index.

Narrow therapeutic index – Drugs with a narrow therapeutic index have a narrow range between their effective dose and toxic dose. Because of this, little variations in plasma concentrations can cause adverse effects or subtherapeutic responses.

The FDA describes these properties for drugs with a narrow therapeutic index:

The difference between the LD_{50} and ED_{50} or between the MEC and MTC is less than two. The drug requires constant patient monitoring and titration.

Examples of drugs with a narrow therapeutic index include:

1. Warfarin
2. Digoxin
3. Digitoxin
4. Levothyroxine
5. Phenytoin
6. Lithium
7. Procainamide
8. Theophylline

9. Cyclosporine
10. Tacrolimus
11. Thiopental
12. Heparin
13. Quinidine
14. Aminophylline
15. Vancomycin
16. Gentamicin
17. Amphotericin B
18. Amikacin
19. Amiodarone
20. Phenobarbital
21. Argatroban
22. Sotalol
23. Everolimus
24. Mycophenolic acid
25. Butriptyline
26. Imipramine
27. Streptomycin
28. Neomycin
29. Diazepam
30. Morphine
31. Ethanol
32. Cocaine

Physical and Chemical Incompatibilities Related to Nonsterile Compounding and Reconstitution

Incompatibility

This is an undesirable or unwanted change that affects the stability, safety, appearance and efficacy of a pharmaceutical product. Incompatibility can occur during the formulation of drugs, compounding, packaging, manufacturing, storage, dispensing and administration. Incompatibility can be therapeutic, chemical or physical.

Physical incompatibility

This occurs when substances are combined in a physical process to yield an undesirable mixture. It is also called pharmaceutical incompatibility. The following are examples of physical incompatibility.

Insolubility – The material does not dissolve into the solvent. The most common causes are the inability of organic and inorganic compounds to dissolve in solvents. Factors that affect solubility include milling, change in pH, chemical reactions, surfactants, co-solvent and complex formation. Common examples of indiffusible solids are zinc oxide, chalk, succinylsulfathiazole, calamine and acetylsalicylic acid. Some tinctures can precipitate when added to an aqueous solution because they contain chlorophyll or resins.

Immiscibility – This occurs when two ingredients are mixed to form a nonhomogenous mixture. Examples are creams, lotions, ointments and emulsions. These drug formulations demonstrate separation and must therefore be stored at room temperature. Causes of immiscibility include incomplete mixing, false time of addition of surfactants, the addition of surfactants with inappropriate concentration, microbial contamination, temperature, mixing oil and water.

Liquefaction – This occurs when solids with low melting points are mixed. In this case, a soft or liquid mass is formed (eutectic mixture). This mixture forms because the melting point of the mixture is reduced until it is below room temperature. Hydrates are then released. It is difficult to compound such mixtures because it is liquid. Examples include menthol, camphor, phenol, aspirin, chloral hydrate and sodium salicylate.

Precipitation – Substances that have been dissolved in a solvent can precipitate if a non-solvent is added. A good example is adding water into an alcoholic solution of resins. Since resins are insoluble in water, they are precipitated. Another example is adding alcohols or salts in high concentrations into aqueous solutions of hydrophilic colloids. This action will precipitate the colloids.

Chemical incompatibility

This occurs when two or more substances are combined to form a mixture that has different chemical properties. In this case, an inactive or toxic product is formed. Causes include the formation of complexes, acid-base hydrolysis, changes in pH, oxidation-reduction changes and double decomposition. These reactions can manifest as decomposition, changes in color, effervescence and explosions.

Types of chemical incompatibility

Based on the chemical interactions:

Tolerated incompatibility – Chemical interactions are caused by changing the order in which the substances are mixed or mixing the substances in their diluted forms. However, the formulation itself is not changed.

Adjusted incompatibility – Incompatibility is caused by adding another substance or substituting one substance for the other.

Based on the nature of the chemical reaction:

Immediate incompatibilities – The reaction occurs after the ingredients are mixed.

Delayed incompatibility – The reaction occurs at a slow rate.

Based on the prescriber:

Intentional – The prescriber intentionally mixes the drugs.

Unintentional – The prescriber unintentionally mixes the drugs because the person does not know they are incompatible.

Therapeutic incompatibility

Therapeutic incompatibility occurs when the therapeutic effect of a drug is modified by another drug. It can be pharmacokinetic or pharmacodynamic.

Dosage error – The most severe form of dosage error is an overdose of medication.

Wrong dose – This involves prescribing a different drug from the one intended. The most common cause is mistaking drugs with similar names (prednisone and prednisolone or digitoxin and digoxin).

Prescribing contraindicated drugs – This occurs when drugs are contraindicated in a patient or disease. For example, cotrimoxazole is contraindicated in patients with reactions to sulfur-containing drugs.

Prescribing synergistic or antagonistic drugs – When two drugs work together to improve the potency of one another, they are synergistic. When they decrease the activity of each other, they are antagonistic.

Drug interactions – This includes drug-drug interactions, drug-food interactions and drug-disease interactions. All these are covered above.

Overview of Body Systems and Their Functions

Anatomy of the circulatory system

The chambers of the heart

Right atrium – The right atrium receives blood from the superior and inferior vena cava. The superior vena cava drains deoxygenated blood from the head, neck and upper limbs, while the inferior vena cava drains deoxygenated blood from the abdomen and lower limbs.

Right ventricle – Blood from the right atrium enters the right ventricle and from there is transported into the lungs via the pulmonary artery.

Left atrium – Oxygenated blood enters into the left atrium via the pulmonary veins.

Left ventricle – Blood from the left atrium enters the left ventricle and then is transported into the systemic circulation via the aorta.

Valves of the heart

The valves of the heart include two atrioventricular valves, which are the tricuspid and bicuspid valves, and two semilunar valves, which are the pulmonic and aortic valves. The heart valves are lined with the endocardium, which is continuous with the chambers of the heart. Also, the heart valves have cusps or flaps that prevent the backflow of blood. The mitral or bicuspid valve has two leaflets and is located between the left atrium and left ventricle. It prevents the backflow of blood into the right atrium during diastole.

The tricuspid valve has three leaflets, the anterior, septal and posterior. It is located between the right atrium and right ventricles and prevents backflow of blood during diastole. The pulmonary valve has right, anterior and left cusps and is located between the right ventricle and the pulmonary trunk. It prevents the backflow of blood into the right ventricle.

The aortic valve is located between the right ventricle and the aorta and prevents the backflow of blood into the right ventricle.

The great vessels of the heart

Superior vena cava

The superior vena cava is a short, large vein that carries deoxygenated blood from the upper limbs, neck and head. The jugular vein, thyroid veins and left and right subclavian veins empty into the superior vena cava. The lymphatic duct drains into the subclavian veins. It is responsible for the circulation of lymph in the plasma.

Inferior vena cava (IVC)

This is the largest vein. It drains deoxygenated blood from the lower limbs, abdomen and pelvis into the heart. It is formed by the confluence of the right and left common iliac veins. The IVC starts posterior to the abdomen in proximity to the aorta in the abdomen. On its way toward the right atrium, the hepatic veins, renal, lumbar and suprarenal veins drain into it.

The aorta
This is the largest artery. Blood from the left ventricle enters the aorta through the aortic valve. The aorta has a large quantity of elastin that makes it sensitive to stretch in response to blood volume and pressure. The aorta expands as the ventricle expels blood through the aortic valve. This pressure is necessary to propel blood and maintain pressure in the diastolic phase. This pressure also creates a pressure gradient in which blood in areas of high pressure flows to areas with low pressure.

Parts of the aorta
The arch of the aorta has baroreceptors and chemoreceptors that respond to changes in pressure, pH and carbon dioxide. Impulses from the chemoreceptors and baroreceptors are transported to the medulla oblongata. The response is then mediated via the sympathetic and parasympathetic nervous systems via the plexus of nerves. From the heart, the aorta travels downward in proximity to the inferior vena cava.

Parts of the aorta include:

The ascending aorta is between the aortic arch and the heart. It branches into the septic sinuses and then forms the coronary arteries.
The arch of the aorta is the highest part of the aorta. It branches into the left subclavian artery, the left carotid artery and the brachiocephalic trunk.
The descending aorta is a component of the aortic arch. It branches into the common iliac arteries, which divide further into the abdominal and thoracic branches of the aorta.
The thoracic part, which is a branch of the descending aorta, divides into the esophageal, mediastinal, esophageal, bronchial and phrenic arteries. The abdominal aorta, which is a branch of the descending aorta, breaks into the iliac arteries and renal and suprarenal arteries. The thoracic aorta is susceptible to aneurysms.

The pulmonary arteries
These arteries transport deoxygenated blood from the right ventricle into the capillaries in the alveoli. These are the only arteries that carry deoxygenated

blood. The right and left pulmonary arteries are wide and short and deliver blood from the lungs to the heart.

The pulmonary veins

Pulmonary veins are the only veins that carry oxygenated blood. Four pulmonary veins open into the left atrium. Together with the pulmonary arteries, they make up the pulmonary circulation.

Anatomy of the peripheral circulation

Arteries – Arteries carry oxygenated blood from the heart to end organs. An artery has three layers. The tunica intima is the innermost layer. It is made of endothelial tissue supported on elastic and fibrous basement membranes. The tunica media is the middle layer of the artery. It is made up of smooth muscles controlled by the autonomic nervous system. These smooth muscles are sensitive to stretch. The tunica adventitia, the outermost layer of the artery, is made of thick connective tissue that binds the artery to surrounding structures.

Veins – Veins carry deoxygenated blood from organs back to the heart. The pressure in veins is less than that in arteries. To facilitate the movement of blood, veins have valves that propel blood upward against gravity.

Arterioles – These are arteries with smaller calibers. They connect arteries to capillaries.
Venules – These are veins with smaller calibers. They connect veins to the capillaries.

Capillaries – These are blood vessels with wide surface areas. Their surface area and endothelium make it easy for nutrients, water and oxygen to diffuse into tissue cells and for carbon dioxide, waste and toxins to be excreted. Capillaries form a network of organs and are connected to arterioles and venules.

Composition of the blood

Blood is a liquid tissue that contains plasma, white blood cells, red blood cells and platelets. These components help blood transport oxygen and nutrients to cells, transport waste and toxins for excretion, form blood clots and control bleeding, fight infection and regulate temperature, hormones and other mechanisms required for homeostasis.

The composition of blood is about 55% plasma (water) and 45% cells. Blood makes up 8% of total body weight. On average, males have about 12 pints of blood while females have about nine pints.

Plasma
Plasma is the liquid component that contains water, protein, sugar, fat and salts. Plasma is a medium for the transportation of blood cells, hormones, nutrients, clotting factors, antibodies, waste products and more.

Red blood cells (also called erythrocytes or RBCs)
Red blood cells are bright red due to their iron content. They are the most abundant cells in the blood and form about 45% of the blood volume. RBCs are biconcave cells with a flat center. This structure makes them pliable and compressible as they pass through arterioles, venules and capillaries.

The production of RBCs is controlled by erythropoietin, a hormone secreted by the kidneys. Erythropoietin stimulates the release and maturation of blast cells in the bone marrow. Because RBCs have no nuclei, they can change shape as they pass through small blood vessels. However, their annucleation gives them a short half-life of about 120 days.
The function of RBCs is the circulation of oxygen. RBCs contain hemoglobin, which readily binds to oxygen molecules and carbon dioxide. Oxygenated blood, which is carried by the arteries (except the pulmonary artery), is bright red. Deoxygenated blood is dark red. Hematocrit is the percentage of red blood cells in the blood volume. It is used to diagnose anemia.

White blood cells
White blood cells are also called leukocytes. Unlike RBCs, white blood cells are fewer in quantity, as they make up 1% of the blood volume. White blood cells protect the body from diseases by fighting bacterial, viral, parasitic and fungal infections. The most common white blood cell is the neutrophil. It makes up 70% of the white blood cell count.

Because neutrophils are the first to respond to infections, they have a very short life span. The second most common white blood cell is the lymphocyte. T lymphocytes confer cellular immunity and mount a direct attack on antigens, while B cells confer humoral immunity and mount an attack via the complement system and antibodies.

Platelets
Platelets are also called thrombocytes. These blood cells are responsible for hemostasis and control of bleeding. They do this by an interplay of clotting factors, inflammatory mediators and growth factors. There are two pathways in which the clotting mechanism is activated. These are the extrinsic (tissue) pathway and the intrinsic pathway. These pathways lead to the activation of thrombin. Thrombin activates fibrin, which in turn polymerizes and forms a platelet plug. A high number of platelets can cause pathologic clotting, while low levels of platelets cause prolonged bleeding.

Physiology of the circulatory system

Cardiac electrophysiology
The cardiomyocytes can depolarize and repolarize. These actions cause generalized and synchronized contractility of the cardiomyocytes.

The heart can generate the initial electrical impulse needed for depolarization. This impulse is generated from the pacemaker cells (the sinoatrial nodes located in the right atrium). The pacemaker initiates the cardiac impulse. This impulse travels to the atria and is transferred to another group of specialized cells called the atrioventricular node (AVN).

The AVN, which is located in the septa between the two atria, conducts impulses from the atria into the ventricles. A delay of about 0.1 seconds allows the ventricles to contract after the atria have contracted, allowing blood in the atrium to empty into the ventricles. From here, the cardiac impulse is transported to the Bundle of His, a group of specialized cells in the ventricles. The right and left branches of the Bundle of His are located in the interventricular septum.

After this, the cardiac impulse is transferred to the apex of the heart via the Purkinje fibers. The impulses are finally shunted to the lateral aspects of the heart.

The arrangement of these cells causes the heart to contract synchronously during systole. On the other hand, the heart muscles relax in a phase called diastole. A cardiac cycle is characterized by atrial systole and atrial diastole and ventricular systole and ventricular diastole.

In the cardiac cycle, the opening and closing of the valves are regulated by the rising and falling of the pressure in the heart chamber. However, the pressure in the left side of the heart is higher than that in the right.

Atrial systole

In this phase of the cardiac cycle, there is a filling of the ventricles. A drop in the pressure in the heart causes blood to flow into the atria. When the atria are filled, the atrioventricular valves are opened, and about 70% of blood flows into the ventricles. This action is passive. When the atrium contracts, the remaining 30% of blood in the atria is ejected into the ventricles.

Ventricular systole

After atrial systole, the blood in the ventricles is called the end-diastolic volume. In ventricular systole, the ventricles contract. Increased pressure causes the aortic and pulmonic valves to open. Blood is then ejected into the pulmonary and systemic circulation.

Isovolumetric relaxation

At the end of ventricular systole, the blood remaining in the ventricles is called the end-systolic volume. The aortic and pulmonic valves close, and pressure in the aorta increases. Meanwhile, the atria go into diastole, fill up with blood and prepare to commence a new cardiac cycle.

Cardiac output

This is the quantity of blood ejected by the heart in one minute. It is calculated by multiplying the stroke volume (quantity of blood ejected by the ventricles in each heartbeat) by the heart rate.

The stroke volume can be calculated by subtracting the ESV from the EDV. Factors that increase stroke volume include exercise, pregnancy, drugs, fever and more.

Frank-Starling law

This principle states that the preload determines the stroke volume. This preload is the quantity of blood that returns to the heart during ventricular filling. Preload is determined by the amount of blood during ejection. This is also called cardiac output. During ventricular filling, the cardiac muscles stretch. This stretching stimulates cardiac contractility and increases cardiac output. This phenomenon shows a positive relationship between preload and cardiac contractility. However, this phenomenon is limited.

Hormones that increase cardiac contractility include thyroxine and adrenaline. These hormones improve the inotropic function of the heart. Calcium channel blockers reduce this function.

Functions of blood

Homeostasis – Blood maintains the internal environment of the body. By transporting water, oxygen, hormones and nutrients and excreting waste and carbon dioxide, blood maintains the osmolality within the intracellular and extracellular space.

Immunologic – Plasma contains immunomodulators—like leukotriene, growth factors and cytokines—needed for cell signaling and immunology. Also, white blood cells respond to antigens and signals from immunomodulators.

Hemostasis – Blood is required for hemostasis and clotting. Plasma contains clotting factors required for coagulation. Also, platelets can aggregate around a ruptured vessel and control bleeding.

Anatomy of the digestive system

Anatomy of the abdomen

The abdomen protects the gut, kidneys and reproductive organs. It is made up of the lumbar spine and muscles that connect the chest to the pelvis.

The lumbar spine has five vertebrae, L1-L5. It makes up the posterior section of the abdomen. These vertebrae are the largest bones in the spinal column and bear weight from the cervical and thoracic spine.

The muscles of the anterior and lateral abdominal wall include the internal and external oblique muscles, transversus abdominis, rectus abdominis and pyramidalis. These muscles act like a girdle that supports the pelvis and lumbar vertebrae and protects the abdominal organs. The muscles of the posterior abdominal wall include the iliacus, quadratus lumborum, diaphragm and psoas minor and major. These muscles work with the anterior abdominal muscles to support the lower spine.

The arteries supplying the anterior and lateral abdominal wall are the superior and inferior epigastric arteries, subclavian artery, musculophrenic artery, posterior intercostal artery, superficial epigastric artery and superficial circumflex iliac artery. The nerves supplying the anterolateral abdominal wall are the iliohypogastric nerve, ilioinguinal nerve, thoracoabdominal, subcostal and lateral cutaneous nerves.

The upper gastrointestinal system

Esophagus – The esophagus starts from the oropharynx and ends at the cardiac part of the stomach. It is a fibromuscular and hollow organ made of stratified squamous epithelium, submucosa, smooth muscle fibers and connective tissue. The lower part of the esophagus, the part opening into the stomach, is made up of simple columnar epithelia.

The esophagus is 25 cm long and located posterior to the trachea, lungs and heart. It opens into the stomach at the level of the diaphragm. The upper part of the esophagus is supplied by the inferior thyroid artery, bronchial arteries and thoracic aorta. The lower part of the esophagus is supplied by the inferior phrenic artery and lower gastric artery. The smooth muscles of the esophagus are controlled by the sympathetic trunk and vagus nerve.

Stomach – The stomach is a hollow organ located in the left hypochondrium of the abdomen. It has two openings. The superior opening connects to the lower end of the esophagus, while the inferior opening connects to the duodenum. Its sole aim is the digestion of swallowed food.

The stomach is lined with simple columnar cells that secrete both gastric acid and mucus. Gastric acid contains hydrochloric acid and pepsin, which are used to digest proteins. The secreted mucus protects the parts of the stomach exposed to gastric acid. Underneath the mucus layer is the submucosal layer consisting of collagen fibers and connective tissue. After this is the muscularis externa, made up of smooth muscles. The serosa is the outermost layer and is continuous with the connective tissue connecting the stomach to other structures. It is also continuous with the peritoneum.

The stomach rests on the spleen, pancreas, transverse colon, left kidney, suprarenal glands and diaphragm. These structures are called the stomach bed. An adult stomach can hold about 2 to 4 L of contents. The greater curvature of the stomach is supplied by the left and right gastroepiploic arteries, while the lesser curvature is supplied by the left and right gastric arteries. The stomach is innervated by the autonomic nervous system.

Small intestine (duodenum) – The duodenum is the first part of the small intestine. It is the shortest segment of the small intestine (about 10 to 15 inches). The superior aperture is a continuation of the pylorus. It is closely related to the biliary tree, the pancreas and the liver. In the duodenum are openings for the pancreatic and bile ducts. These ducts carry digestive enzymes for digesting fats and carbohydrates. The enzymes also increase the pH of digested food. The duodenum is supplied by the gastrointestinal and superior mesenteric arteries. It is innervated by the autonomic nervous system.

The lower gastrointestinal system

Jejunum – This is the second part of the small intestine. Its main purpose is absorbing nutrients from digested food. It is about 2.5 m in length. The mucosa of the jejunum contains lots of villous processes with increased surface area for quick absorption via passive diffusion.

Ileum – This is the last segment of the small intestine. It is a place where bile salts, cobalamin and other nutrients (not absorbed by the jejunum) are absorbed. The ileum opens into the colon via the ileocecal valve.

Large intestine – This includes the cecum, colon, rectum and anus. The large intestine is a place for the absorption of water and the formation of solid/semisolid feces. It is about 1.5 m long. The large intestine begins from the ileocecal valve and ends at the anus. Chyme from the ileum enters the cecum, goes into the ascending colon, then the transverse colon, then goes down into the descending colon and is stored in the rectum. Apart from absorbing water and salts, bacterial flora located in the large intestine ferment the parts of the chyme that cannot be digested. The large intestine is supplied by both the superior and inferior mesenteric arteries. These arteries are innervated by the splanchnic plexus of nerves.

Accessory organs

Liver – The liver is the primary organ for the metabolism of nutrients. It is a highly vascularized organ located in the right hypochondrium and epigastrium of the abdomen. It secretes bile, a digestive juice needed for digestion of fat and alkalinization of digested food. This bile juice is stored and concentrated in the gallbladder. It weighs about 1.5 kilograms.

The functional unit of the liver is the lobule. Each liver lobule is made up of millions of hepatocytes. These lobules are surrounded by capillaries called sinusoids. The liver is supplied by the hepatic artery and hepatic vein and is in close relation with the inferior vena cava.

Pancreas – The pancreas is a retroperitoneal organ located underneath the stomach and the left lobe of the liver. It has both endocrine and exocrine functions. The exocrine function is the secretion of digestive juices and enzymes like amylase, used in digesting carbohydrates; lipase, used in digesting fat; trypsin, used in digesting protein; phospholipase; and cholesterol esterase. The endocrine function of the pancreas includes the secretion of hormones like insulin, glucagon, somatostatin and pancreatic polypeptide.

Gallbladder – This is a small, hollow organ located underneath the right lobe of the liver. It receives bile juice from the liver via the common hepatic duct. Once received, bile juice is stored and concentrated and then moved into the duodenum via the common bile duct. Bile is used for the emulsification of fats, making them easy to absorb.

Physiology of the digestive system

Digestion – The primary function of the digestive system is the digestion of complex compounds into simple absorbable nutrients. This is made possible via the action of digestive juices, enzymes and bacteria on food. From the mouth, salivary juices contain maltase, which breaks down carbohydrates. Saliva also moistens and softens food, making it easy to swallow. In the stomach, hydrochloric acid coagulates protein and activates pepsinogen to form pepsin. Pepsin, in turn, breaks down protein into amino acids. In the duodenum, bile secreted via the bile duct emulsifies fat and, along with pancreatic juices, increases the alkaline content of the chyme. The pancreas secretes amylase, lipase and trypsinogen used to digest carbohydrates, fats and proteins.

Absorption – Absorption mainly starts from the duodenum and continues at the ileum and colon. As stated earlier, the jejunum has villous processes with a large surface area. Here, glucose, vitamins, fatty acids and amino acids are absorbed via passive diffusion. In the colon, water, salts and bile acids are absorbed.

Metabolic – The liver is responsible for most metabolic functions in the body. This is because, under the influence of insulin, glucose is stored in the liver as glycogen. Excess glycogen is stored in muscles. Excess glycogen is converted into fatty acids and stored in the adipose tissue. The liver also metabolizes amino acids to form plasma B cells, thrombopoietin and clotting factors (including antithrombin, protein S and protein C). Apart from proteins, the liver metabolizes fatty acids, alcohol, drugs and toxins.

Endocrine – The pancreas secretes hormones like insulin and glucagon, which are used for the metabolism of carbohydrates, amino acids and fatty acids. The pancreas also secretes somatostatin and pancreatic polypeptide, hormones required for peristalsis and the secretion of pancreatic juices. The enterochromaffin cells in the liver secrete small quantities of serotonin, substance P and motilin.

Hematologic – In the embryonic stage, the liver is used for erythrogenesis. Although this function is lost by 32 weeks, the liver acts as a reservoir for venous blood. Apart from this, since the liver metabolizes clotting factors, it is required for hemostasis. Intrinsic factor, which is found in the stomach, binds with cobalamin and makes it absorbable. In the gut, bacterial flora act on food and stimulate the metabolism and absorption of vitamin K. Vitamin K is required to activate vitamin K–dependent clotting factors.

Excretion – The liver is involved in the metabolism of drugs and toxins. In the gut, particularly the large intestine, feces are excreted along with microbes, cholesterol and excess salt.

Immunologic – The liver is responsible for the formation of plasma proteins from amino acids. It also has Kupfer cells, which are phagocytes involved in the mononuclear phagocytes system. In the gut, Peyer's patches are nests of lymphoid tissue in the small intestine. These lymphoid tissues are responsible for secreting IgA, a secretory immunoglobulin used to control the proliferation and colonization of gut flora.

Anatomy of the endocrine system

Hypothalamus – The hypothalamus is a small gland located beneath the thalamus. It is a component of the limbic system. The hypothalamus has three regions in the sagittal plane—the mamillary, supraoptic and tuberal regions—and three areas in the coronal plane—the medial, periventricular and lateral areas. In the anterior region, there is the preoptic nucleus, which controls temperature; the medial preoptic nucleus, which secretes GnRH; the supraoptic nucleus, which releases vasopressin and oxytocin; the paraventricular nucleus, which releases oxytocin, TRH, CRH and vasopressin; the anterior hypothalamic hormones, which inhibit thyrotropin and control sweating, panting and temperature; and the suprachiasmatic nucleus, which controls the circadian rhythm.

The tuberal region contains the dorsomedial hypothalamic nucleus (heart rate, blood pressures stimulation of the gastrointestinal tract), the ventromedial nucleus (satiety, neuroendocrine function), the arcuate nucleus (hunger, GHRH, inhibition of prolactin) and the lateral nucleus.

The mammillary region contains the mammillary nucleus (for memory), lateral nucleus, posterior nucleus (blood pressure, release of vasopressin, dilation of pupils), and tuberomammillary nucleus (arousal, sleep, memory and feeding.)

Pituitary gland – This is a pea-sized endocrine gland located below the hypothalamus. It is divided into anterior, middle and posterior regions. The anterior pituitary contains lactotrophs (secrete prolactin), somatotropes (secrete growth hormone), gonadotropes (secrete gonadotropic hormones), corticotrophs (secrete adrenocorticotropic hormone), and thyrotropes (secrete thyroid-stimulating hormone). The middle part of the globe secretes melanocyte-stimulating hormone, while the posterior part of the globe is connected to the hypothalamus by the pituitary stalk.

Thyroid gland – This is a butterfly-shaped gland located in the anterior part of the neck. The thyroid gland contains follicular cells that secrete thyroxine (T4), triiodothyronine (T3) and calcitonin. The secretion of these hormones is dependent on feedback from thyroid-stimulating hormone from the anterior pituitary and thyrotropin-releasing hormone from the hypothalamus. The thyroid gland is supplied by the superior thyroid artery (from the external carotid artery) and the inferior thyroid artery (from the thyrocervical trunk). It is controlled by the autonomic nervous system. Sympathetic innervation is from the cervical trunk, while parasympathetic innervation is from the recurrent and superior laryngeal nerve.

Parathyroid glands – There are four parathyroid glands located at the back of the thyroid gland. These glands secrete the parathyroid hormone. The parathyroid glands are supplied by the superior and inferior thyroid arteries. They are also innervated by the middle and inferior cervical ganglion.

Pancreas – The pancreas is a retroperitoneal organ located underneath the stomach and the left lobe of the liver. It has both endocrine and exocrine functions. The endocrine function of the pancreas includes the secretion of hormones like insulin, glucagon, somatostatin and pancreatic polypeptide.

Testes – This is the primary reproductive organ in males. The testes secrete testosterone. The secretion of testosterone is controlled by the gonadotropin-releasing hormone via the hypothalamus and the follicle-stimulating hormone and luteinizing hormones from the anterior pituitary. The testes are supplied by the testicular arteries, cremasteric artery and artery to the ductus deferens.

Ovaries – The ovaries are the primary reproductive organs in females. They produce and release ova. The ovaries secrete progesterone, estrogen, testosterone and inhibin. The release of these hormones is controlled by gonadotropin-releasing hormone via the hypothalamus and follicle-stimulating hormones, and luteinizing hormones from the anterior pituitary. The ovaries are supplied by the external and internal iliac arteries.

Suprarenal glands – These glands are found on top of the kidneys. The adrenal cortex has three layers: the zona reticularis, the zona glomerulosa and the zona fasciculata. The zona reticularis releases androgens. The zona fasciculata releases cortisol, and the zona glomerulosa releases aldosterone. The adrenal medulla releases catecholamines. The adrenal glands are highly vascularized by the superior, inferior and middle suprarenal arteries.

Pineal gland – This is a reddish-gray gland located in the midbrain. It is a part of the epithalamus. This gland secretes melatonin, a hormone that controls sleep-wake cycles and circadian rhythm. It is supplied by the posterior cerebral artery.

Physiology of the endocrine system

Thyrotropin-releasing hormone – This hormone is released from the hypothalamus. It stimulates the release of thyroid-stimulating hormone from the anterior pituitary.

Corticotropin-releasing hormone – This hormone is released from the hypothalamus. It stimulates the release of ACTH from the anterior pituitary.

Gonadotropin-releasing hormone – This hormone is released from the hypothalamus. It stimulates the release of follicle-stimulating and luteinizing hormones from the anterior pituitary.

Thyroid-stimulating hormone – This hormone is released from the anterior pituitary. It stimulates the release of T4 and T3 from the thyroid.

Adrenocorticotropic hormone – This hormone is released from the anterior pituitary. It stimulates the release of cortisol from the adrenal glands.

Follicle-stimulating hormone (FSH) – This hormone is secreted from the anterior pituitary. In both males and females, FSH activates the maturity of primordial germ cells. In mature males, it maintains spermatogenesis, while in mature females, it stimulates the follicular phase of the menstrual cycle.

Luteinizing hormone – This hormone is secreted by the anterior pituitary. In mature females, it stimulates the production of estradiol. It also triggers ovulation. In pubertal males, it encourages the secretion of testosterone from the Leydig cells.

Thyroxine – This hormone is secreted from the follicular cells in the thyroid glands. Thyroxine is responsible for maintaining metabolism in the body. Some of its metabolic functions include metabolic rate, digestion, heart rate, brain function and bone metabolism. The thyroid, anterior pituitary and hypothalamus form a TRH-TSH-thyroxine feedback mechanism.

Parathyroid hormone – This hormone is released by the parathyroid glands. It is responsible for bone metabolism and the metabolism of vitamin D, calcium and phosphate.

Calcitonin – This hormone is released by the thyroid glands. It has an inhibitory effect on the parathyroid hormone.

Aldosterone – This hormone is released by the zona glomerulosa of the adrenal cortex. It is responsible for water and electrolyte metabolism and balance.

Cortisol – This hormone is released from the zona fasciculata of the adrenal cortex. Functions of cortisol include calcium metabolism, glucose metabolism, immunomodulation, electrolyte and water metabolism and blood pressure control. The hypothalamus, pituitary and adrenal cortex form a CRH-ACTH-cortisol feedback mechanism.

Catecholamines – This includes epinephrine and norepinephrine. These hormones are released from the adrenal medulla. They are responsible for initiating sympathetic activity.

Estrogen – Estrogen is released from the ovaries. This hormone is responsible for the follicular phase of the menstrual cycle in mature females. During puberty, estrogen is responsible for the proliferation and maturation of the alveoli tissue in the breast, deposition of fat in the hips and buttocks, and feminization.

Progesterone – This hormone is secreted by the corpus luteum during ovulation. It stimulates and sustains vascularization of the endothelium in anticipation of pregnancy. If implantation does not occur, a decline in progesterone causes shedding of the endometrium.

Testosterone – Testosterone is secreted by the testes. However, small quantities of androgens are secreted by the cells in the zona reticularis of the adrenal cortex. During puberty, testosterone causes masculinization. In mature adults, it stimulates the production of sperm in the testes.

Prolactin – This hormone is secreted in the anterior pituitary. Prolactin stimulates lactogenesis during and after pregnancy. It also drives the milk let-down reflex. Prolactin has inhibitory actions on progesterone and estrogen.

Oxytocin – This hormone is secreted by the hypothalamus and released by the posterior pituitary. Oxytocin is the main driver of uterine contractions during labor. Oxytocin also drives the milk let-down reflex. This hormone stimulates maternal instincts and encourages bonding between a mother and an infant.

Vasopressin – This is also called antidiuretic hormone. It is produced in the hypothalamus and secreted by the posterior pituitary. Vasopressin acts on the cells in the collecting tubules of the nephrons, stimulating the absorption of water. This action concentrates urine.

Growth hormone – This hormone is secreted by the anterior pituitary. It is responsible for the growth of long bones, muscles and other somatic cells.

Glucagon – This hormone is secreted by the alpha cells in the pancreas. Glucagon stimulates the release of glucose from glycogen and fatty acids during a fasting state.

Insulin – This hormone is secreted by the beta cells in the pancreas. Insulin stimulates the conversion and storage of glucose as glycogen and fatty acids, which are then stored in the liver, adipose tissue and skeletal muscle cells. Under the influence of insulin, amino acids are also stored in muscle cells and used to repair worn-out muscles.

Melatonin – This hormone is released by the pineal gland. It controls sleep-wake cycles. It is also an antioxidant used to mop up free radicals and therefore reduces oxidative stress.

Anatomy of the skin

The skin has three layers—the epidermis, dermis and hypodermis.

Epidermis – This is the superficial layer of the skin that protects the other layers from friction, heat and other extreme physical factors. The epidermis is made up of stratified squamous epithelial (keratinocytes). The epidermis is not vascularized and depends on the dermis and hypodermis for nutrients and water. The epidermis also contains melanocytes, which are pigment-containing cells that protect the skin from UV radiation.

Dermis – The dermis is thicker than the epidermis. It is vascularized and contains blood vessels, hair follicles, nerves and sweat glands. It is rich in collagen and elastin fibers and is responsible for keeping the skin turgid and firm.

Hypodermis – This is the deepest layer of the skin. It is largely made up of subcutaneous fat, which is stored for insulation, cellular support and energy consumption.

Physiology of the skin

Protection – The epidermis protects the body from mechanical forces that can be injurious. It also protects the body from dehydration, microorganisms, infection, thermal factors and UV radiation.

Sensory – The skin is innervated by a rich supply of nerves that receive, transmit, interpret and act on tactile stimuli.

Thermoregulation – The hypodermal layer of the skin contains subcutaneous fat that insulates the body from cold. Also, this layer acts as an energy reservoir when the food supply is low.

Biochemistry – The skin is involved in lots of biochemical functions required to maintain homeostasis, such as synthesizing vitamin D required for calcium and phosphorus metabolism.

Anatomy of the lymphatic system

Lymphatic organs

Spleen – The spleen is a solid organ located in the left hypochondrium, just underneath the diaphragm and stomach. It is supplied by the splenic artery and splenic vein. It is innervated by the splenic plexus of nerves from the vagus nerve and celiac ganglia. The spleen has an outer layer called the red pulp and an inner layer called the white pulp. The red pulp has blood-filled sinusoids that filter red blood cells and store monocytes. The white pulp is responsible for its lymphatic function. It has nodules made of lymphoid follicles and T lymphocytes. These nodules are called Malpighian corpuscles.

Thymus – This is a pinkish lobulated tissue located in the neck. After puberty, it is slowly involuted and replaced by fatty tissues. The thymus has two regions. The outer region is the cortex. This area is rich in T lymphocytes. The inner medullary area is rich in epithelial tissues and Hassall's corpuscles. It also has some quantities of lymphocytes. The thymus is supplied by the anterior intercostal arteries and internal costal arteries. It is innervated by the autonomic nervous system.

Red bone marrow – The red bone marrow is rich in progenitor stem cells that can differentiate to become white blood cells, platelets or red blood cells. Red bone marrow is found in spongy bones.

Lymphatic vessels

Superficial vessels – These are found in the subcutaneous layer of the skin and course along with veins. They drain into the deep lymphatic vessels.

Deep vessels – These vessels drain the organs in the body and course along with the arteries. Lymph in lymphatic channels drains into lymphatic vessels and moves toward the right lymphatic duct and thoracic duct via the lymph nodes. The right lymphatic duct drains the upper right side of the body, that is the right upper limbs, right hemithorax and right side of the head and neck. The thoracic duct, which is bigger than the right lymphatic duct, drains the other side of the body. The two ducts eventually empty into the subclavian veins.

Lymphatic nodes

Lymph nodes are bean-shaped glands that filter the plasma/lymph. There are about 450 lymph nodes in the body, most of which are found in the abdomen. Each lymphatic node has B lymphocytes, T lymphocytes and other cells. If there are offending antigens in the plasma, an immune response is triggered. More inflammatory cells are recruited into the nodes. This phenomenon causes nodes to swell up during infection. Lymph fluid enters the node via the afferent channel and leaves the nodes via the efferent channels.

Lymphatic fluid – Lymphatic fluid is a transudate. It is transparent and yellowish. Lymph is formed when fluid moves from capillaries into tissue spaces. This movement is initiated by the high hydrostatic pressure in the arterioles. Lymph is very similar to plasma. About 95% of lymph is made of water. The other

5% consists of lipids, proteins, carbohydrates and lymphocytes. Chyle, which is lymph from the gastrointestinal tract, is rich in fatty acids.

Physiology of the lymphatic system

Immunologic – The primary function of the lymphatic system is immunologic. White blood cells—which are formed in the spleen, thymus and red bone marrow—are mobilized into the lymph nodes. As lymph flows into the lymph nodes, it is filtered by these white blood cells. Thus, filtration is necessary before the lymph flows into the heart.
Hemostasis – By absorbing excess plasma in the tissue space, the lymphatic system maintains a balance of fluid between the intracellular and extracellular spaces.
Excretion – The lymphatic system helps filter out abnormal cells that are too big to drain into the venules and enter the venous circulation. In the lymph nodes, these cells are ingested by phagocytes.

Anatomy of the muscular system

Striated muscle – The functional unit of striated muscle is the sarcomere. It is found between two Z lines. Under a microscope, these sarcomeres appear as light and dark bands that alternate with each other. The sarcomere is made of two proteins. Actin makes up the thick filament, while myosin makes up the thin filament. The head of the myosin filament binds to actin filament. This occurs when actin binds to calcium. The groups of myofibrils from muscle fibers.

Groups of muscle fibers form fascicles. Groups of fascicles form skeletal muscle. There are over 650 striated muscles in the body. These muscles make up 40% of body weight. Skeletal muscles are innervated by the somatic nervous system. Skeletal muscles, unlike cardiac and smooth muscles, are multinucleated.

Smooth muscle – Unlike skeletal muscles, smooth muscles are nonstriated and involuntary muscles. These muscles do not contain sarcomeres. Instead, they are arranged as single-unit or multi-unit muscles. Single-unit muscles stretch or relax as a whole. These muscles are found in the muscles of the gut, urinary tract and blood vessels. Multi-unit muscles found in the trachea and iris stretch/relax in part. The functional unit of the muscle is the myocyte. It is a spindle-shaped cell with tapered ends and wide bodies. These cells do not contain myofibrils. However, there are actin and myosin filaments in the cytoplasm that make the myofibrils sensitive to stretch and contraction.

Cardiac muscle – Cardiac muscles are striated involuntary muscles. These muscles are found only in the heart. Just like the skeletal muscle, the functional unit of cardiac muscle is the sarcomere. However, unlike skeletal muscle, the impulse for contraction is generated by specialized cardiac cells called the Purkinje cells. These cells generate currents that pass through the cardiac muscle. Because the sarcomeres are connected by intercalated discs, muscle contraction and relaxation are synchronized.

Physiology of skeletal muscles

The motor unit of skeletal muscle initiates the contraction of the sarcomere. The motor unit is made up of the motor neuron and its afferent and efferent fibers. When stimulated by the motor neuron, the muscle fibers are depolarized. During depolarization, acetylcholine is released at the neuromuscular junction. Acetylcholine then stimulates the release of calcium. Calcium binds to actin and stimulates muscle contraction.

Physiology of smooth muscle

The contraction of smooth muscles can be spontaneous or caused by external factors. Smooth muscles in the gut can contract spontaneously via pacemaker cells of Cajal. The contraction of smooth muscles can also be influenced by drugs, hormones and neurotransmitters released from the autonomic nervous system.

During contraction, the myosin and actin filaments slide over each other. ATP drives this action. However, unlike skeletal and cardiac muscles, smooth muscles do not depend on the binding of calcium on troponin. Instead, calcium regulates the phosphorylation of myosin.

Physiology of cardiac muscles

The physiology of cardiac muscles is covered under cardiac electrophysiology.

Anatomy of the nervous system

Anatomy of the brain

The cerebrum – This is the largest part of the brain. The cerebrum is divided into the right and left hemispheres. The corpus callosum, a bundle of fibers, connects the two hemispheres. The cerebrum is divided into the front lobe, temporal lobe, parietal lobe and occipital lobe.

The cerebrum is also divided into the diencephalon and the telencephalon. The telencephalon is made up of the basal nuclei, subcortical fibers and cerebral cortex. The diencephalon is made up of the hypothalamus and thalamus.

The cerebral cortex is the outermost layer of the cerebrum. It is gray and therefore called gray matter. The cortex has a wrinkled appearance to increase surface area. These wrinkles are called gyri, while the grooves between the gyri are called sulci. Myelinated axons located underneath the gray matter have a white appearance. This part of the cortex is called white matter.

The basal nuclei are made up of the putamen, substantia nigra, globus pallidus and subthalamic nucleus. The putamen and globus pallidus make up the lentiform nuclei, while the putamen and caudate nucleus make up the striatum.

The thalamus relays input into the cortex. It is made up of nuclei, including the anterior nuclei, ventrolateral nuclei, lateral nuclei and the lateral and medial geniculate bodies. The hypothalamus is found in the third ventricle, just underneath the thalamus. It is made up of nuclei that secrete hormones and enzymes responsible for maintaining homeostasis.

The brain stem – The brain stem is made up of the medulla oblongata, pons and midbrain. The medulla oblongata is continuous with the cervical spinal cord. It is made up of pyramids, gracile tubercles and cuneate tubercles. Also, the roots of the XII, IX and X cranial nerves emerge.

The pons is on top of the medulla. The pons is made up of pontocerebellar fibers that project from corticopontine fibers. The VI, VII and VIII cranial nerves emerge from the pons. The midbrain is the most superior part of the brain stem. From it, the III and IV cranial nerves emerge.

The cerebellum – The cerebellum is in the posterior fossa of the skull. It has a wrinkled appearance for an increased surface area. The cerebellum has two hemispheres connected by a vermis.

Anatomy of the meninges

The meninges include the pia mater, arachnoid mater and dura mater. The pia mater is the innermost layer. It adheres to the gyri and sulci of the cortex. The middle layer is the arachnoid mater. Between the pia and arachnoid mater is the subarachnoid space, which contains CSF. The dura mater is the outer layer. This layer adheres to the inferior aspect of the skull. The meningeal dura is continuous with the brain, while the periosteal dura is continuous with the skull. The subdural space is found between the arachnoid and dura mater.

Anatomy of the spinal cord

The spinal cord begins from the medulla and ends at the L1-L2, which is the upper part of the lumbar vertebrae. It tapers into the conus medullaris and ends into a vertical sheaf, forming the cauda equina. The white matter of the spinal cord contains both ascending and descending myelinated tracts. These tracts convey both sensory and motor impulses. The gray matter is located in the central part of the spinal cord and is H-shaped. It is made up of non-myelinated fibers and cell bodies.

At the anterior horn of the gray matter are lower motor neurons that conduct impulses through the descending corticospinal tracts. The axial part of these neurons acts as efferent fibers. The anterior horns of the gray matter carry sensory fibers that come from the dorsal root ganglia. In the gray matter are also neurons that transmit sensory, motor and reflex impulses from the dorsal nerve roots to the ventral nerve roots from one part or level of the spinal cord to the other. The spinothalamic tracts carry pain and temperature impulses in the contralateral side of the spinal cord, while most of the other tracts carry impulses on the ipsilateral side of the spinal cord. There are 31 pairs of nerve roots in the spinal cord.

Physiology of the nervous system

Cranial nerves

There are 12 cranial nerves.

I – The olfactory nerve is responsible for smell.

II – The optic nerve is responsible for sight.

III – The oculomotor nerve is responsible for eye movement and mediating the pupillary reflex.

IV – The trochlear nerve is responsible for moving the superior oblique muscle.

V – The trigeminal nerve has both motor and sensory functions. The ophthalmic and trigeminal divisions of this nerve receive sensory input from the eyes and face. The last division, the mandibular nerve, gives motor function to the muscles of mastication.

VI – The abducens give motor function to the lateral rectus nerve.

VII – The facial nerve gives motor function to the muscles of facial expression. It also gives sensory function to the tongue and ear.

VIII – The vestibulocochlear nerve gives hearing and vestibular function to the ear.

IX – The glossopharyngeal nerve gives the tongue taste sensation and sensation of touch to the oropharynx. It is responsible for the gag reflex.

X – The vagus nerve gives parasympathetic function to the gut and heart.

XI – The accessory nerve gives motor innervation to the trapezius and sternocleidomastoid muscles.

XII – The hypoglossal nerve gives motor function to the muscles of the tongue.

Cerebral cortex

The frontal lobe controls reasoning, speaking, attention and other higher functions. The parietal lobe controls visuospatial interpretation, language, comprehension, awareness and proprioception. The occipital lobe controls visual comprehension and perception. The temporal lobe controls auditory perception, visual and verbal memory and language.

Thalamus

The thalamus relays visual and auditory stimuli to the cortex. The substantia nigra is responsible for controlling body movement.

Hypothalamus

The hypothalamus regulates functions responsible for homeostasis (endocrine function and regulation, temperature control, hunger, thirst and sleep).

Amygdala

The amygdala controls emotions (such as fear, sexual desire and anger) and memory.

Hippocampus

It is responsible for creating memories and nostalgia.

The cerebellum

The cerebellum controls posture, movement, balance and cardiac and respiratory function.

Brain stem

The brain stem controls vital functions like heart rate, respiratory rate and blood pressure.

Anatomy of the reproductive system

The male reproductive system

External genitalia

The external genitalia include the penis and the scrotum. The penis has a long shaft and a glans penis. The shaft of the penis is made up of spongy tissues that fill up with blood during arousal. The penis is supplied by the pudendal artery. The scrotum is inferior to the penis. It houses the testicles. When the temperature is low, the cremaster muscle contracts, pulling the scrotum into the abdomen. The dartos muscle also contracts, increasing the rugae on the scrotum. The scrotum is connected to the pelvic cavity via the inguinal canal. The spermatic cord (which contains the spermatic artery, spermatic vein and nerve) passes through the inguinal canal.

The internal genitalia

The internal genitalia are made up of the testis, epididymis, vas deferens and other accessory glands. The testis produces sperm and synthesizes testosterone in the Leydig cells. The epididymis is a place for the transport and maturation of sperm. The vas deferens channels the sperm cells from the epididymis to the ejaculatory duct. Accessory glands include the prostate gland, seminal vesicles and Cowper glands.

The female reproductive system

Female external genitalia

The female external organ is the vulva. The vulva is made of the pudendal cleft, mons pubis, Bartholin's gland, clitoris, labia majora and minora and vaginal introitus.

Female internal genitalia

This includes the vagina, cervix, uterus, fallopian tubes and ovaries.

Physiology of the reproductive system

The actions of hormones on the reproductive system are covered in the physiology of hormones. During copulation, arousal causes an erection of the penis. At climax, semen moves from the epididymis. It is ejaculated from the ejaculatory duct as it gets to the seminal tubules. Sperm cells in the semen ascend toward the cervix. During ovulation, a single ovum is released from the ovaries. It enters the fallopian tube and is fertilized by a sperm cell. After fertilization, the fertilized ovum becomes a morula. This morula implants into the endometrium of the uterus.

Anatomy of the respiratory system

Anatomy of the chest

The chest is made up of the thoracic spine, ribs, muscles, fat, neurovascular bundles and skin. It protects the heart, lungs and liver and supports the upper extremities and shoulders. Even if the thoracic spine is bony, its connection to muscles makes it flexible enough to permit expansion of the chest wall during inspiration.

The surface landmarks of the anterior chest wall include the sternal notch and nipple. The midsternal line is measured from the sternal notch to the xiphoid process. The landmark of the lateral sternal line is down the lateral border of the sternum. It is used in locating the internal thoracic artery. The midclavicular line is identified from the middle part of the clavicle down to the medial side of the nipple. This landmark is used in performing a thoracostomy.

The superior boundaries of the axilla include the outer part of the first rib, the superior part of the scapula and the middle third part of the clavicle. The lower border of the axilla makes up the inferior boundary. The anterior border is made up of the pectoralis major and minor, while the posterior border is made up of the latissimus dorsi. The anterior axillary line, which is used in placing a chest tube, is drawn from the anterior axillary border down to the chest wall. The posterior axillary line is drawn down from the posterior axillary border to the chest. The midaxillary line is drawn from the apex of the axilla.

The skeleton of the thorax is made up of 12 thoracic vertebrae (T1-T12) (posterior aspect), 12 pairs of ribs (lateral and anterior) and a sternum (medial and anterior). The first seven ribs are called true ribs because they attach to the manubrium and sternum. The eighth, ninth and tenth ribs are called false ribs because their costal cartilages join together to connect to the sternum through the costal arch. The eleventh and twelfth ribs are called floating ribs. The sternum is made of three bones: the manubrium, sternal body and xiphoid process. The sternum acts as a pivot for the attachment of muscles. The muscles of the chest wall include the intercostal muscles, which move the ribs, the transversus thoracis, the pectoralis major and minor, and serratus anterior.

The neurovascular structures are located in the inferior border of each rib in the costal groove. During thoracentesis and thoracostomy, the costal space is entered via the superior border. The ribs are nourished by the intercostal branches of the internal thoracic artery (a branch of the subclavian artery). The anterior chest wall is innervated by the medial and lateral pectoral nerves (branches of the brachial plexus).

The upper airway – The upper airway is made up of the nasal cavity, the pharynx and the larynx. During inspiration, air goes from the nose into the nasal cavity. In the nasal cavity, the air is humidified and dust particles are filtered by nasal hairs. Humidified air currents move into the pharynx and then into the larynx. The entrance of the larynx is guarded by the epiglottis, which prevents food passage into the lower respiratory tract.

The lower airway – The lower airway is made up of the trachea and bronchi. Air flows from the trachea and into the carina, then into the main bronchi. From the main bronchi, it moves into the alveoli in the bronchioles, which are highly vascularized tissues that allow the exchange of oxygen for carbon dioxide.

The lungs are protected by the rib cage. Below the lungs is the diaphragm, a fibromuscular structure that separates the lungs from the abdominal organs. The diaphragm is also an accessory muscle for inspiration. It is controlled by the autonomic branch of the nervous system.

The lungs are further protected by the pleura, a fibrous sac that encloses the lungs. The inner layer of the pleura is called the visceral pleura; it lubricates the lungs and reduces friction. It also provides nutrients and oxygen to the lungs. The outer layer is called the parietal pleura. It is tough and fibrous and protects the lungs from injury.

Physiology of the respiratory system

During inspiration, the diaphragm increases intrathoracic pressure by becoming flat and pulling the ribs outward and upward. The lung expands, and air flows into the nasal cavity and down to the alveoli in the bronchioles. The alveoli are made up predominantly of Type 1 pneumocytes, squamous cells that allow the exchange of carbon dioxide for oxygen. During exhalation, the diaphragm shortens back to its initial length. This causes the chest cavity to return to its original size and allows the expulsion of air through the nose.

Oxygen in the alveolar capillaries is carried via the hemoglobin in red blood cells into the systemic circulation. At tissue spaces, oxygen is uncoupled from hemoglobin and diffuses into the cells. Carbon dioxide diffuses from the tissue into the capillaries and venous circulation.

Anatomy of the skeletal system

Axial skeleton – This consists of the skull, ribs, sternum and vertebrae.

Appendicular skeleton – This includes the bones of the upper and lower limbs. There are about 213 bones in the human body. Of these, 74 are in the axial skeleton, 126 bones are in the appendicular skeleton, and six bones are the auditory ossicles.

Types of bone

Compact bone – This is also called cortical bone. This bone is dense and strong and is found in long bones (diaphysis).

Cancellous bone – This is also known as woven bone. This bone is not as dense as compact bone and has loose lattices. This bone is found in the metaphyses and epiphyses of long bones.

Bones are grouped into:

Long bones – Radius, ulna, clavicle, humerus, femur, fibula, tibia, metatarsal and phalanges

Short bones – Tarsals, carpals, patella, sesamoids

Irregular bones – Sacrum, hyoid bone, coccyx and vertebrae

The parts of a long bone include:

Diaphysis – This is the central part of the shaft of the bone. It is made of cortical bone tissue and is often called the isthmus.

Metaphysis – This is the part of the bone between the diaphysis and epiphysis. It is made up of cancellous bone.

Epiphysis – This is the growing end of the bone in children. In adults, it is the remaining part of the growth plate.

Medullary cavity – This cavity is within the long bone. It is rich in bone marrow.

Periosteum – This is the outer part of bone tissue. It has nerve fibers and blood vessels that nourish the bone. It also has osteoblasts and osteoclasts.

Anatomy of the urinary system

Kidneys

The kidneys are bean-shaped solid retroperitoneal organs located in the lumbar region. The adrenal glands are on top of the kidneys. The kidneys and the adrenal glands are covered by perirenal fat. This fat is located between the renal fascia and renal capsule. The kidneys have two regions, the cortex and the medulla. The renal cortex is the outermost portion of the kidney and is located between the renal capsule and renal medulla.

In adults, the cortex forms an outer zone called cortical columns that extends into the pyramids. The renal cortex contains renal corpuscles and tubules. The renal medulla is the inner part of the kidney. It is divided into renal pyramids. Here, the renal arteries divide into the interlobar arteries. These arteries divide into arcuate arteries and form the interlobular arteries. The interlobular arteries form the glomerulus.

Ureters – The ureters transport urine from the kidneys into the bladder. In adults, ureters are about 30 cm long. The epithelium of the ureter is the transitional epithelial. The smooth muscles in the ureters promote peristalsis.

Bladder – This is a hollow organ that stores urine from the ureters. The adult bladder can hold about 300 to 500 mLs of urine.

Urethra – The urethra transports urine from the bladder to the urethral meatus. In males, it is about 20 cm in length, while in females, it is about 4 cm in length.

Physiology of the renal system

The nephron is the functional unit of the kidneys. It is made up of a renal corpuscle and a renal tubule. The renal corpuscle is made up of the glomerulus and bowman's capsule. The renal tubule is made up of the loop of Henle and proximal and distal convoluted tubules. There are about 1.5 million nephrons in an adult.

Blood enters the glomerulus via the afferent arterioles and leaves by the efferent arterioles. The diameter of the afferent arterioles is smaller than that in the efferent arterioles. This causes hydrostatic pressure in the glomerulus that drives ultrafiltration. The ultrafiltrate passes through the loop of Henle and proximal and distal convoluted tubules. As it passes, water and ions are reabsorbed or excreted depending on the osmolality of the blood. Filtrates like urea and creatinine are excreted and never reabsorbed.

Anatomy of the eye

Sclera – This is the outermost layer of the eye. It is avascular and protects the eye.

Choroid – This is the middle layer of the eye. It is highly vascularized and provides nutrients and oxygen to the retina and sclera of the eye. It also replenishes the aqueous and vitreous humor of the eye.

Retina – This is the innermost layer of the eye. It is highly innervated and is responsible for sending light impulses to the brain via the optic nerve.

Cornea – This is responsible for transmitting and focusing light into the retina.

Lens – This directs light to the retina. Its size is controlled and adjusted by the ciliary body.

Ciliary body – This is a muscle that helps control the shape of the lens. It is posterior to the iris.

Iris – This is the pigmented part of the eye. It controls the amount of light that reaches the retina.

Pupil – This is located in the center of the iris. Its size is controlled by the oculomotor nerve. It adapts to the intensity of light entering the eye.

Macula – This is located in the retina. It has specialized light-sensitive cells. It degenerates as we age.

Fovea – The center area of the macula is responsible for sharp vision.

Optic nerve – This is a bundle of nerve fibers coming from the retina. It transmits light impulses to the occipital part of the cerebral cortex.

Vitreous humor – This is a gelatinous substance that keeps the eye globular. It fills up the center part of the eye.

Physiology of the eye

Light waves enter the eye through the cornea. The cornea is responsible for refracting the light waves into the iris. From the iris, light enters the lens and is ultimately focused on the retina. The retina transfers this light energy into electrical impulses that are transmitted via the optic nerve to the occipital lobe of the brain for interpretation.

Anatomy of the ear

The outer ear is composed of the auricle, external auditory meatus and tympanic membrane. The middle ear is made up of the tympanic cavity, which contains the auditory ossicles and the epitympanic recess. The inner ear is made up of the vestibule, cochlea, semicircular canals and membranous labyrinth.

Physiology of the ear

Sound waves are collected by the pinna and channeled into the ear canal. On arriving in the tympanic membrane, the sound waves cause a vibration of the ear ossicles, which amplifies the sound waves. These sound waves are directed into the bony and membranous labyrinth and are converted into electrical impulses. The electrical impulses are directed to the temporal lobe via the vestibulocochlear nerve.

Anatomy of the nose

The external nose is made of the nasal bone and lateral nasal cartilages. The internal part of the nose consists of the nasal septum. The nasal septum is made up of the superior, inferior and middle turbinates; the lacrimal duct; and the sinuses. The epithelia of the nasal mucosa are the ciliated pseudostratified columnar epithelial. The cilia filter humidified air from the duct and direct mucus toward the nasopharynx. The nose is supplied by the external and internal carotid arteries.

Physiology of the nose

As air enters the nose, it is humidified and filtered from dust particles. The mucus in the nose acts as an immunologic defense against microbes. The nose is an organ for smell. The mucosa of the upper nasal canal has Bowman's glands that help in generating impulses for smell. These impulses are transmitted to the frontal lobe via the olfactory nerve.

Anatomy of the tongue

The tongue is a muscle covered by specialized epithelia. It is divided into three regions: the tip, body and base. The median sulcus divides the tongue into right and left halves, while the terminal sulcus separates the body of the tongue from its base.

The tongue has four intrinsic and four extrinsic muscles. The intrinsic muscles include the superior and inferior longitudinal muscles and the vertical and transverse muscles. These muscles change the tongue's shape. The extrinsic muscles are the palatoglossus, hyoglossus, styloglossus and genioglossus muscles. These muscles change the tongue's position.

Physiology of the tongue

The surface of the tongue is covered with papillae, which contain taste buds, specialized cells for taste. These taste buds can detect sour, sweet, salty and umami. These papillae include the fungiform, valate and foliate papillae.

Chapter 3: Overview of Drugs

Drugs for the Cardiovascular System

Antihypertensive drugs

Adrenergic agonists – Adrenergic agonists stimulate alpha 2 adrenergic receptors in the brain stem and reduce the activity of the sympathetic nervous system. Side effects include depression, drowsiness and lethargy. Examples include clonidine, methyldopa and guanfacine.

Angiotensin-converting enzyme inhibitors – Angiotensin-converting enzyme inhibitors prevent the conversion of angiotensin I to angiotensin II (which releases bradykinin, causes vasoconstriction and stimulates the release of aldosterone). These drugs reduce resistance in peripheral vessels without causing reflex tachycardia. Side effects include dry cough and angioedema, which is a potential and serious side effect. These drugs also increase potassium and creatinine levels. Examples are captopril, enalapril, lisinopril and fosinopril.

Angiotensin II receptor blocker – These drugs inhibit the stimulation of angiotensin II receptors and therefore inhibit activation of the Renin-angiotensin system. Angiotensin receptor blockers should not be used together with an ACEI. They are useful in hypertensive patients with diabetic nephropathy. Examples include telmisartan, losartan, valsartan and candesartan.

Calcium channel blockers – Calcium channel blockers prevent the action of calcium on smooth muscles and therefore reduce resistance in peripheral blood vessels. Examples are dihydropyridines, including amlodipine, nifedipine, felodipine and nicardipine. The nondihydropyridines reduce heart rate, myocardial contractility and atrioventricular conduction. They are not used in patients with atrioventricular blocks caused by left ventricular failure. Examples are verapamil and diltiazem.

Diuretics – Diuretics reduce preload by reducing plasma volume. Examples are loop diuretics, like furosemide and torsemide. They are potassium-sparing diuretics. Thiazide-type diuretics include hydrochlorothiazide, chlorothiazide, hydroflumethiazide and indapamide. These diuretics are potassium-wasting diuretics and cause hypokalemia. Potassium-sparing diuretics include amiloride and spironolactone. Side effects of these drugs are hyperkalemia, gynecomastia (spironolactone), nausea and GIT disturbances.

Direct vasodilators – Direct vasodilators work directly on peripheral blood vessels without affecting autonomic nervous system activity on the blood vessels. Examples are hydralazine and minoxidil. Side effects include tachycardia, headaches and edema. These drugs increase the risk of angina in patients with coronary artery disease.

Nitrates – Nitrates are potent vasodilators that reduce afterload. Examples are sodium nitroprusside and nitroglycerin. Side effects include rebound hypertension, reflex tachycardia and postural hypotension. These drugs must not be taken with phosphodiesterase 5 inhibitors (sildenafil).

Antiplatelets

COX-2 inhibitors – COX-2 inhibitors bind to the serine residue on COX-2 and irreversibly inhibit the action of COX-2 in initiating platelet aggregation. Examples are aspirin, triflusal, salsalate and choline magnesium trisalicylate. Side effects include nausea, abdominal pain, flatulence and diarrhea. Others are tinnitus, blurred vision, gastrointestinal bleeding, water retention and kidney failure.

ADP receptor inhibitors – ADP receptor inhibitors bind to and irreversibly inhibit the P2Y12 receptor. This action reduces cAMP and prevents activation of glycoprotein IIb/IIIa receptors required for platelet aggregation. Examples are prasugrel, clopidogrel and ticlopidine. Side effects include bleeding, rashes, nausea and diarrhea.

Glycoprotein IIB/IIIA inhibitors – Glycoprotein IIB/IIIA inhibitors bind to glycoprotein IIb/IIIa receptors and prevent binding of fibrinogen. This action prevents aggregation of platelets. Examples are eptifibatide, tirofiban and abciximab. Side effects include bleeding, bradycardia and hypotension.

Thromboxane inhibitors – Thromboxane inhibitors both prevent the action of thromboxane synthase and block thromboxane receptors. Examples include antagonists of thromboxane receptors (ifetroban and dipyridamole) and thromboxane synthase inhibitors like picotamide. Side effects include bleeding.

Thrombolytics

Streptokinase – This binds to plasminogen and facilitates its conversion into plasmin. Plasmin breaks down fibrin and fibrinogen in blood clots. Side effects include bleeding from the gums, fever, rashes, hypotension, flushing and allergic reactions.

Recombinant tissue plasminogen activators – These are enzymes that facilitate the conversion of plasminogen to plasmin. Plasmin breaks down fibrin and blood clots. Examples are alteplase, tenecteplase and reteplase. Side effects include bleeding, particularly hemorrhagic stroke. Others are allergic reactions, thromboembolism, shock sepsis, pulmonary edema and angioedema.

Anticoagulants

Warfarin – Warfarin inhibits the synthesis of vitamin K–dependent clotting factors (factors II, X, IX and VII). It also inhibits the actions of protein Z, C and S and proteins like matrix Gla protein and osteocalcin. Side effects include bleeding, which can manifest as intracranial hemorrhage and hemorrhagic stroke. Other side effects include flatulence, cramps, nausea, vomiting and allergic reactions.

Heparin – Heparin binds to antithrombin III and hastens its inhibitory action on factor Iia and factor Xa. It also inhibits factors XII, IX, plasmin and XI. Side effects include bleeding, allergic reactions, abdominal cramps, bloating and flatulence, purple toe syndrome and chest pain.

Factor Iia/Xa inhibitors – Iia inhibitors directly inhibit the action of thrombin and prevent coagulation. Xa inhibitors work by inhibiting the action of factor Xa. Examples of Iia inhibitors include dabigatran, argatroban, lepirudin and hirudin. Examples of Xa inhibitors include apixaban, betrixaban, rivaroxaban and fondaparinux. Side effects include bleeding and allergic reactions.

Antiarrhythmics

Class I (sodium channel blockers) – Class I sodium channel blockers block the transport of sodium ions and increase refractoriness, reduce automaticity, conduction velocity and repolarization. Examples of Class Ia include disopyramide, quinidine and procainamide. Class Ib includes lidocaine and phenytoin. Class Ic includes encainide and flecainide. Side effects include constipation, dry mouth, blurred vision, urinary retention, headaches and tachycardia.

Class II (beta-blockers) – Class II beta-blockers block sympathetic activity and decrease heart rate without affecting blood pressure. Examples are atenolol, esmolol, propranolol, metoprolol and timolol. Side effects include bradycardia, hypotension, hypoglycemia, hyperglycemia, difficulty breathing (bronchoconstriction), depression, dizziness and fatigue.

Class III (potassium channel blockers) – Class III potassium channel blockers inhibit sympathomimetic action, increase action potential, reduce AV and SA node conduction and increase repolarization. Examples include sotalol, amiodarone, bretylium, betapace and dronedarone. Side effects include bradycardia, heart block, blue skin syndrome (amiodarone), photosensitivity, constipation, photodermatitis, dizziness and hepatotoxicity.

Class IV (calcium channel blockers) – Class IV calcium channel blockers block calcium influx and increase SA and AV nodal repolarization. They also reduce myocardial contraction. Examples are verapamil, diltiazem and isoptin. Side effects include constipation, hypotension, edema, nausea, rashes and headaches.

Class V (others) – Examples include digoxin, adenosine and magnesium sulfate.

Diuretics

Loop diuretics – Loop diuretics act on the sodium-potassium-calcium transporter (NKCC2) in the thick ascending limb of the loop of Henle. They prevent the reabsorption of sodium, potassium and chloride. Examples are furosemide, ethacrynic acid, torsemide and bumetanide. Side effects include hyponatremia, hypomagnesemia, hypokalemia, hyperuricemia/gout, syncope, postural hypotension, metabolic alkalosis, tinnitus, dyslipidemia, ototoxicity, deafness and allergic reactions.

Thiazides – Thiazides inhibit the reabsorption of sodium and chloride ions in the distal convoluted tubules. They also enhance the reabsorption of calcium ions in the distal convoluted tubules. Examples are chlorothiazide, hydrochlorothiazide, indapamide and chlorthalidone. Side effects include hypokalemia, hypomagnesemia, hypercalcemia, hyperglycemia, hyperlipidemia, hyperuricemia/gout and hypocalciuria.

Aldosterone antagonists – Aldosterone antagonists inhibit the action of aldosterone and prevent excretion of potassium and reabsorption of sodium in the distal and collecting tubules. Examples are spironolactone and eplerenone. Side effects include polyuria, diarrhea, stomach cramps, hyperkalemia and gynecomastia.

Drugs for the Central Nervous System

Analgesics

NSAIDs – These drugs bind to the serine residue on COX and inhibit the action of COX, an enzyme that acts on the formation of prostaglandins, thromboxanes and other inflammatory mediators. NSAIDs can be selective or nonselective. Nonselective inhibitors include salicylates, like aspirin, triflusal, salsalate and choline magnesium trisalicylate; propionic acid derivatives, like ibuprofen, ketoprofen and naproxen; acetic acid derivatives, like sulindac, indomethacin and diclofenac; and COX-2 inhibitors, like celecoxib, firocoxib, parecoxib and lumiracoxib. Common side effects include nausea, abdominal pain, flatulence and diarrhea. Others include tinnitus, blurred vision, gastrointestinal bleeding, water retention and kidney failure. Nonselective COX inhibitors increase the risk for gastrointestinal bleeding and kidney failure.

Acetaminophen – This is a mild nonselective COX inhibitor. Paracetamol is an example. Side effects include nausea, abdominal cramps, gastrointestinal bleeding, allergic reactions and the risk for Reye's syndrome.

Opioids – These stimulate the opioid receptors in the CNS. Examples are alkaloids like morphine and codeine, derivatives of alkaloids like hydrocodone, buprenorphine, oxycodone and hydromorphone, and synthetic opioids like pethidine, methadone, diphenoxylate, loperamide, pentazocine, butorphanol, levomethorphan and tramadol.

Withdrawal symptoms are anxiety, tachypnea, diaphoresis, lacrimation, yawning, rhinorrhea, diarrhea, anorexia, tremors, fever, tachycardia, hypertension and stomach cramps. Symptoms are usually not fatal. Overdose symptoms are respiratory depression, apnea, miosis, hypotension, delirium, bradycardia, hypothermia and urinary retention.

Anticonvulsants

Benzodiazepines – These drugs stimulate GABA receptors. When these receptors are activated, chloride channels are opened. Examples are diazepam and midazolam.

Barbiturates – These drugs stimulate GABA secretion by binding to receptors located on chloride ion channels. By binding to them, they keep chloride ion channels opened longer. Examples are phenobarbital and methylphenobarbital.

Sodium channel blockers – These drugs block the sodium channels in neuronal membranes. The action is dose dependent because antagonism works only in therapeutic doses. Examples are phenytoin, lamotrigine, carbamazepine and lacosamide.

Calcium channel blockers – These drugs block the flow of calcium into the neuronal membranes. Examples are ethosuximide, gabapentin, pregabalin and valproic acid.

Those acting on glutamate synapses and other actions – Drugs like levetiracetam reduce the release of glutamate by binding to carrier proteins. Felbamate blocks glutamate NMDA receptors. Perampanel blocks the AMPA receptors. Phenobarbital also blocks glutamate receptors.

Side effects of antiseizure drugs

Benzodiazepines – Tolerance, sedation and dependence

Carbamazepine – Teratogenicity, ataxia, Stevens-Johnson syndrome, drowsiness, induces hepatic enzymes and blood dyscrasia

Ethosuximide – Headaches, lethargy and gastrointestinal distress

Felbamate – Liver failure and aplastic anemia

Gabapentin – Nystagmus, sedation and ataxia

Lamotrigine – Dizziness, Stevens-Johnson, rash, ataxia and nausea

Levetiracetam – Psychosis, hallucinations, weakness and sedation

Perampanel – Induce CYP enzymes, headaches, somnolence and behavioral changes

Phenobarbital – Somnolence, tolerance and dependence and induction of hepatic enzymes

Phenytoin – Gingival hyperplasia, hirsutism, peripheral neuropathy, nystagmus and induces hepatic enzymes

Retigabine – Somnolence, discoloration of retina and skin and dysarthria

Tiagabine – Asthenia, nausea and abdominal pain

Topiramate – Drowsiness, paresthesia and memory impairment

Valproic acid – Weight gain, hair loss, tremor and nausea

Vigabatrin – Dizziness, weight gain and sedation

Zonisamide – Dizziness, diarrhea, rash, weight loss, confusion and Stevens-Johnson syndrome

Antiparkinsonian agents

Dopaminergics

Levodopa – Levodopa crosses the blood-brain barrier and has a higher bioavailability than endogenous dopamine. It is converted to dopamine by the enzyme dopa decarboxylase. Side effects include dyskinesia, gastrointestinal effects like nausea and vomiting, cardiovascular effects like postural hypotension, asystole and tachycardia, and behavioral changes like agitation, hallucinations, delusion and psychosis.

Carbidopa – Carbidopa increases the bioavailability of levodopa in the brain by inhibiting the actions of dopa decarboxylase in peripheral tissues. Side effects are the same as levodopa.

Amantadine – Amantadine stimulates dopaminergic activity in the neurons by either increasing dopamine reuptake or increasing secretion of dopamine. The mechanism is, however, unclear. Side effects include behavioral changes, like agitation, hallucinations, delusion and psychosis. It can also cause urinary retention, gastrointestinal upset, peripheral edema and postural hypotension.

Dopamine agonists – These drugs stimulate dopamine receptors. Examples are pramipexole, a non-ergot and a D3 receptor agonist; ropinirole, a D2 receptor agonist and a non-ergot; and bromocriptine, a D2 receptor partial agonist and an ergot alkaloid. Side effects include dyskinesia, gastrointestinal effects like nausea and vomiting, cardiovascular effects like postural hypotension, asystole and tachycardia, and behavioral changes like agitation, hallucinations, delusion and psychosis. Bromocriptine also causes pulmonary infiltration and erythromelalgia.

Monoamine oxidase inhibitors – These drugs inhibit monoamine oxidase B, an enzyme that breaks down dopamine. Examples are rasagiline, selegiline and safinamide. Side effects include hypotension, dyskinesias, insomnia, changes in mood and gastrointestinal distress. High risk for serotonin syndrome when used with SSRIs.

Catechol-O-methyltransferase (COMT) inhibitors – These drugs inhibit COMT, an enzyme that metabolizes methyldopa into 3-O-methyldopa (3-OMD), a competitive substrate with levodopa. Examples are tolcapone and entacapone. Side effects include postural hypotension, dyskinesias and gastrointestinal distress. They also cause orange discoloration of the urine and insomnia.

Anticholinergics – These block muscarinic receptors in the CNS and reduce neuronal excitability. Examples are biperiden, benztropine and orphenadrine. Side effects include hallucinations, delusions, confusion, tardive dyskinesia and peripheral effects.

Antipsychotics

Antipsychotics block dopamine receptors (D2) in the hypothalamus, nucleus accumbens, caudate-putamen and cerebral cortex. Second-generation antipsychotics also block receptors, like the alpha-adrenergic receptors, 5-HT2 receptors, H1 and D4 receptors. These antipsychotics have a lesser risk for extrapyramidal effects. Examples of first-generation antipsychotics are chlorpromazine, haloperidol, fluphenazine, trifluoperazine and thioridazine. Second-generation antipsychotics, also known as atypical antipsychotics, include clozapine, quetiapine, olanzapine, ziprasidone and risperidone.

Side effects

Neurologic effects – Dose dependent and reversible. Include rigidity, bradykinesia, tremors, dystonia and akathisia. These effects are more likely with haloperidol and other first-generation antipsychotics.

Tardive dyskinesias – Can be irreversible, very common with first-generation antipsychotics.

Autonomic effects – Caused by antagonism of alpha-adrenergic receptors and muscarinic receptors in peripheral tissues. Symptoms are antimuscarinic effects, like urinary retention, dry mouth, constipation and blurry vision. Blockade of M receptors causes confusion and delusion. Blockade of alpha-adrenergic receptors causes postural hypotension and delayed ejaculation.

Endocrine and metabolic effects – Caused by blockade of dopaminergic receptors. Symptoms are hyperprolactinemia, weight gain and hyperglycemia.

Neuroleptic malignant syndrome – Caused by extrapyramidal effects of mostly first-generation antipsychotics. Symptoms are hyperpyrexia, muscle rigidity and autonomic symptoms.

Sedation – Common with second-generation antipsychotics that block histamine receptors (phenothiazines).

Bipolar agents

Lithium

The mechanism of action is not well established. It inhibits enzymes involved in the formation of phosphoinositides. Phosphoinositides are used to make messengers responsible for the transmission of neuroamines. Side effects include ataxia, sedation, tremor, aphasia, goiter, hypothyroidism, nephrogenic diabetes insipidus, leukocytosis, edema and weight gain.

Antidepressants

Tricyclic antidepressants (TCAs) – TCAs inhibit the reuptake of norepinephrine and serotonin in the brain. Examples are imipramine, amitriptyline and clomipramine. Side effects include fatigue, sedation, somnolence and confusion. Sympathomimetic symptoms are sweating, tachycardia, insomnia and agitation. Other symptoms are postural hypotension, weight gain, paresthesias, tremors and cardiomyopathy.

Selective serotonin reuptake inhibitors (SSRIs) – SSRIs prevent the reuptake of serotonin. They can also mildly inhibit the reuptake of norepinephrine and mildly antagonize adrenergic and cholinergic receptors. Examples are escitalopram, sertraline, fluoxetine, fluvoxamine and paroxetine.

Side effects include nausea, anxiety, headaches, sexual dysfunction and agitation. They can also cause extrapyramidal symptoms, like dystonic reactions, dyskinesias and akathisias. Withdrawal symptoms are anxiety, dizziness, tremor and palpitations. Some drugs can inhibit certain hepatic enzymes and increase the bioavailability of drugs. Serotonin syndrome occurs when an SSRI is taken with an MAOI, muscle relaxants, TCAs, St John's wort, MDMA, meperidine and dextromethorphan.

Serotonin-norepinephrine reuptake inhibitors – Serotonin-norepinephrine reuptake inhibitors prevent the reuptake of serotonin and norepinephrine. Unlike TCAs, they do not inhibit muscarinic, histamine (H1) and alpha-adrenergic receptors. Examples are venlafaxine and duloxetine

Serotonin 5-HT2 antagonists – Serotonin 5-HT2 antagonists block 5-HT2 receptors. Examples are trazodone and nefazodone.

Monoamine oxidase inhibitors – Monoamine oxidase inhibitors disrupt the metabolism of norepinephrine and serotonin at the nerve endings. Examples are phenelzine, tranylcypromine and selegiline. Side effects include hypertensive crisis when taken with food that contains high amounts of tyramine (cured meats, fermented milk, fermented soy milk, cheeses, red wine, dry sherry, pickled vegetables, etc.). The risk of serotonin syndrome is high if taken with SSRI.

Heterocyclics – Mirtazapine inhibits alpha 2 adrenergic receptors and thereby increases the release of norepinephrine and serotonin from nerve endings. The mechanism of action of bupropion is not known. Examples are bupropion, amoxapine and mirtazapine.

Side effects of SNRIs, heterocyclics and serotonin 5-HT2 antagonists

Side effects include weight gain and sedation. Mirtazapine, trazodone and maprotiline can cause autonomic symptoms. Amoxapine blocks dopamine receptors and can cause amenorrhea, galactorrhea, parkinsonism and akathisias. Bupropion causes dry mouth, dizziness, agitation, anxiety and psychosis. Venlafaxine increases blood pressure and withdrawal symptoms.

Anxiolytics, sedatives and hypnotics

Benzodiazepines – Benzodiazepines stimulate GABA receptors. When these receptors are activated, chloride channels are opened. Examples are diazepam and midazolam. Side effects include tolerance, sedation and dependence.

Barbiturates – Barbiturates stimulate GABA secretion by binding to receptors located on chloride ion channels. By binding to them, they keep chloride ion channels opened for longer. Examples are phenobarbital and methylphenobarbital. Side effects include somnolence, tolerance, dependence and induction of hepatic enzymes.

Cholinergics

Direct-acting cholinergics – Direct-acting cholinergics stimulate nicotinic and muscarinic receptors. Examples are acetylcholine, nicotine and pilocarpine.

Indirect-acting cholinergics – Indirect-acting cholinergics bind to acetylcholinesterase and prevent degradation of acetylcholine. Examples are organophosphates, edrophonium and carbamates.

Side effects – Stimulation of muscarinic receptors causes bronchoconstriction, miosis, urinary frequency, salivation, diarrhea, tearing, abdominal cramps and vasodilation. Other symptoms are bradycardia, reflex tachycardia, nausea and vomiting. Stimulation of nicotinic receptors causes CNS stimulation characterized by agitation, restlessness and convulsions. This is then followed by CNS depression.

Anticholinergics

Acetylcholine receptor antagonists – Acetylcholine receptor antagonists block the muscarinic or nicotinic receptors. Examples are atropine, which is an example of a muscarinic antagonist and hexamethonium and mecamylamine, which are examples of nicotinic antagonists.

Side effects – Features of atropine toxicity include hyperpyrexia, dryness of the mouth and eyes, tachycardia, constipation, acute urinary retention and blurry vision. Other symptoms include amnesia, sedation, hallucinations, delirium, flushing and heart block.

Adrenergics

Direct-acting adrenergics – Direct-acting adrenergics directly stimulate alpha or beta receptors or both. Examples are nonselective adrenergic agonists, like norepinephrine; alpha-receptor agonists, like phenylephrine; alpha 2 receptor agonists, like clonidine; nonselective beta-agonists, like isoproterenol; beta 1 adrenergic agonists, like dobutamine; and beta 2 adrenergic agonists, like albuterol.

Indirect-acting adrenergics – Indirect-acting adrenergics inhibit the reuptake of adrenaline (cocaine). Amphetamine stimulates the release of adrenaline. These drugs do not readily pass the BBB, so they have limited CNS effects. Adverse peripheral effects are cardiac arrhythmias, vasoconstriction, pulmonary edema, hemorrhagic stroke and bleeding. Alpha-1-agonists cause hypertension, while beta 2 agonists cause tremors of the skeletal muscle. Beta 1 agonists cause arrhythmias and tachycardia.

Adrenergic antagonists

Adrenergic antagonists antagonize alpha and beta-adrenergic receptors. Examples include irreversible nonselective blockers like phenoxybenzamine, reversible nonselective blockers like phentolamine, selective alpha 1 blockers like prazosin, selective alpha 2 blockers like yohimbine, nonselective beta-blockers like propranolol, beta 1 blockers like atenolol, and beta 2 blockers like butoxamine.

Drugs for the Endocrine System

Hypothalamic and pituitary drugs

Growth hormone agonists – Somatropin and mecasermin

Growth hormone antagonists – Pegvisomant and octreotide

GnRH agonists – Gonadorelin

GnRH antagonists – GnRH receptor antagonists like ganirelix and GnRH receptor agonists like leuprolide

Prolactin antagonists – D2 receptor agonists (bromocriptine)

Oxytocin agonist – Oxytocin

Vasopressin agonists – Desmopressin

Vasopressin antagonists – Conivaptan

Thyroid and antithyroid drugs

Thyroid drugs

Levothyroxine (T4)/Liothyronine (T3) – These drugs have the same functions as endogenous T3 and T4. T3 is more potent than T4. Toxicity resembles hyperthyroidism and thyrotoxicosis (palpitations, heat intolerance, moist skin, diarrhea, tremors, nervousness, polyphagia) and increased deep tendon reflexes.

Antithyroid drugs

Thioamides – Thioamides inhibit the synthesis of thyroxine by blocking the action of peroxidase and blocking iodination. They also block the conversion of T4 to T3. Examples are propylthiouracil and methimazole. Side effects include agranulocytosis, rashes, vasculitis, hepatitis and hypoprothrombinemia.

Iodide and iodine – They block the iodination of tyrosine and release of thyroid hormone. They also decrease blood flow to the thyroid gland. An example is Lugol's iodine. Side effects include metallic taste, drug fever, rash, anaphylaxis and coagulopathy.

Anion inhibitors – They block iodine uptake by antagonizing the iodide transporter. Examples are perchlorate and thiocyanate. Side effects include unstable results and aplastic anemia.

Gonadal hormones and blockers

Estrogens – An example is ethinyl estradiol. The risk for toxicity depends on the dose. When used in pubertal girls, the risk for dwarfism is high due to the early closure of epiphyseal plates. Other adverse effects include risk for breast cancer, endometrial cancer, stroke, myocardial infarction, deep vein thrombosis, hypertriglyceridemia, migraine headaches, gallbladder disease and hypertension. Diethylstilbestrol (DES) increases the risk of ectopic pregnancy, vaginal adenocarcinoma and infertility in female fetuses.

Anti-estrogens – Includes aromatase inhibitors, receptor antagonists like tamoxifen and fulvestrant, and GnRH agonists like danazol.

Progestins – Includes L-norgestrel. Long-term use increases the risk of osteoporosis. Other effects include high blood pressure and decreased high-density lipoprotein.

Antiprogestin – An example is mifepristone, which works by preventing the impact of progesterone

Androgens – Includes testosterone. When used on females, it causes virilization characterized by deepened voice, enlarged clitoris, menstrual abnormalities and hirsutism. Toxicity in males causes feminization characterized by gynecomastia, infertility and shrinkage of the testes. High doses in both sexes increase the risk of cholestatic jaundice and liver cancer.

Anti-androgens – Includes androgen receptor antagonists like flutamide, 5α-reductase inhibitors like finasteride, synthesis inhibitors like ketoconazole, and others, like GnRH agonists, estrogens and progesterone.

Antidiabetic drugs and insulins

Biguanides – Biguanides block renal and hepatic gluconeogenesis. They also stimulate glycolysis in peripheral tissues, uptake of glucose, reduce glucose absorption in the GIT and reduce plasma levels of glucagon. An example is Metformin. Side effects include gastrointestinal symptoms like diarrhea and nausea and lactic acidosis, particularly in alcoholic patients and patients with liver or renal disease.

Insulin secretagogues – Insulin secretagogues stimulate the release of endogenous insulin by facilitating the closure of K+ channels in the beta cells. Examples are sulfonylureas like tolbutamide, second-generation sulfonylureas (glimepiride), glipizide and glyburide. Others include repaglinide, nateglinide and meglitinide. Adverse effects are hypoglycemia, particularly with first-generation sulfonylureas, allergic reactions and weight gain.

Thiazolidinediones – Thiazolidinediones increase tissue sensitivity to insulin by stimulating the peroxisome proliferator–activated receptor-gamma nuclear receptor (PPAR-f receptor). Examples include pioglitazone and rosiglitazone. Side effects include heart failure, edema and anemia. Rosiglitazone increases the risk of myocardial infarction. Troglitazone and pioglitazone induce cytochrome P450 enzymes and reduce the bioavailability of cyclosporine and oral contraceptives.

Glucagon-like peptide-1 (GLP-1) – GLP-1 stimulates the release of insulin from the beta cells, slows down gastric emptying and inhibits the secretion of glucagon. Examples are exenatide, albiglutide, liraglutide and dulaglutide. Side effects include GI disturbances, acute pancreatitis and hypoglycemia.

Dipeptidyl peptidase-4 (DPP-4) inhibitors – DPP-4s inhibit dipeptidyl peptidase-4 (DPP-4), an enzyme that metabolizes GLP-1. Examples are sitagliptin, linagliptin, saxagliptin and vildagliptin. Side effects include headaches, anorexia and nasopharyngitis.

Alpha-glucosidase inhibitors – Alpha-glucosidase inhibitors inhibit alpha-glucosidase, an enzyme responsible for converting complex sugars to monosaccharides. This action reduces postprandial hyperglycemia. Examples are miglitol and acarbose. Side effects include abdominal pain, flatulence, diarrhea and hypoglycemia.

Pramlintide – Pramlintide activates receptors responsible for the control of serum glucose and osteogenesis. It also slows down the rate of gastric emptying and blocks the release of glucagon. Side effects include gastrointestinal symptoms and hypoglycemia.

Sodium-glucose transporter 2 (SGLT2) inhibitors – SGLT2s block reabsorption of glucose. This causes glucosuria. Examples are dapagliflozin, canagliflozin and empagliflozin. Side effects include urinary tract infections and hypotension.

Insulin – Insulin has the same effects as endogenous insulin. Examples are rapid-acting insulin (insulin aspart), insulin lispro and insulin glulisine. Short-acting insulin (insulin regular), intermediate-acting insulins (NPH insulin), long-acting insulins (insulin determine), insulin glargine and insulin degludec. Side effects include hypoglycemia, allergic reactions and hypertrophy of subcutaneous tissue.

Drugs for the Respiratory System

Antiasthmatic drugs and drugs for COPD

Beta adrenoceptor agonists – Beta adrenoceptor agonists activate beta receptors in the smooth muscles and trigger bronchodilation. Examples are albuterol, salmeterol, terbutaline and metaproterenol. Side effects include tremors of skeletal muscles and tachycardia. Arrhythmias can occur if they are used for long.

Methylxanthines – Methylxanthines inhibit the action of phosphodiesterase (PDE), an enzyme that breaks down vAMP to AMP. By blocking this enzyme, they increase concentrations of cAMP, which initiates relaxation of smooth muscle. Examples are theophylline, caffeine and theobromine. Side effects include insomnia, tremor and gastrointestinal problems. Symptoms of toxicity are nausea, hypotension, cardiac arrhythmias and seizures.

Muscarinic receptor blockers – Muscarinic receptor blockers block the muscarinic receptors in the smooth muscles of the bronchial tree. This action prevents bronchoconstriction. Examples are ipratropium, aclidinium, tiotropium and umeclidinium. Side effects include mild symptoms of atropine poisoning.

Corticosteroids – Corticosteroids block the synthesis of arachidonic acid, an inflammatory mediator precursor, by inhibiting the enzyme phospholipase A2 and COX-2. Examples are inhalational corticosteroids like dexamethasone, fluticasone, flunisolide, budesonide and beclomethasone. Inhalational corticosteroids increase the risk of oral and pharyngeal candidiasis. Systemic corticosteroids increase the risk of Cushing's syndrome characterized by weight gain, striae, skin atrophy, hypertension, hyperglycemia and fungal infections of the skin, among others.

Leukotriene antagonists – Leukotriene antagonists drugs block the production and action of leukotriene, an immunomodulator responsible for chemotaxis.
Examples are antagonists of leukotriene receptors (zafirlukast and montelukast). Another example is Zileuton, which inhibits the synthesis of lipoxygenase. Another example is cromolyn, which prevents the release of leukotriene and histamine from mast cells. Side effects of leukotriene receptor antagonists are allergic reactions like granulomatous angiitis. However, the risk for adverse effects and toxicity is low. Side effects of zileuton include hepatitis and elevated liver enzymes. The side effects of cromolyn include drug allergies and cough.

Anti-IgE antibodies – Anti-IgE antibodies are monoclonal and prevent the release of inflammatory mediators from mast cells activated by IgE antibodies. Examples are omalizumab, benralizumab, reslizumab and mepolizumab.

Side effects include immunosuppression with increased risk for respiratory and gastrointestinal infections.

Drugs for the Gastrointestinal System

Drugs for peptic ulcers

Antacids – Antacids neutralize stomach acid by binding with protons in the gut. They also stimulate secretory properties of the gut mucosa. Examples are aluminum hydroxide, magnesium hydroxide, sodium bicarbonate and calcium bicarbonate. Magnesium hydroxide causes diarrhea, while aluminum hydroxide causes constipation.

H2-receptor antagonists – H2-receptor antagonists prevent the production of gastric acid by blocking the histamine 2 receptors in the gastric cells. Examples are cimetidine, famotidine, ranitidine and nizatidine. Cimetidine induces and inhibits certain cytochrome p450 enzymes. Because of this, cimetidine has interactions with more than a hundred drugs. Other side effects of cimetidine are gynecomastia, confusion in geriatric patients, dizziness, headaches and gastrointestinal symptoms.

Proton pump inhibitors – Proton pump inhibitors are irreversible antagonists of the H+/K+ ATPase receptors in the parietal cells. Examples are omeprazole, lansoprazole, pantoprazole and rabeprazole. Side effects include headache, diarrhea and abdominal pain. Chronic use increases the risk of hypergastrinemia.

Sucralfate – Sucralfate forms polymers that bind to erosions and peptic craters. Because it is not absorbed, the risk for adverse effects is insignificant.

Misoprostol – Misoprostol acts like endogenous prostaglandin E1 and stimulates secretion from mucosa glands. It also blocks the secretion of gastric acid. Side effects include diarrhea and other gastrointestinal symptoms; it has a risk for abortion.

Colloidal bismuth – Colloidal bismuth forms a protective layer on ulcers and erosions. It also has antimicrobial properties. A side effect is the formation of tarry stools.

Laxatives

Bulk laxatives – Bulk laxatives promote peristalsis by bulking stools up with insoluble fiber. Examples are psyllium, polycarbophil and methylcellulose. Side effects include gastrointestinal distress (bloating, cramps and flatulence). Bulk laxatives are not to be used in patients with intestinal obstruction or fecal impaction, elderly and debilitated patients and patients with difficulty swallowing.

Stimulant laxatives – Stimulant laxatives stimulate peristalsis by irritating the gut mucosa. Examples are senna, bisacodyl, sodium picosulfate and glycerol. Side effects include abdominal cramps, vomiting, diarrhea, nausea and tolerance. These laxatives are not to be used in patients with severe dehydration, fecal impaction and inflammatory bowel disease.

Osmotic laxatives – Osmotic laxatives pull fluid into the lumen of the gut and stimulate peristalsis. Examples are magnesium hydroxide, sorbitol, lactulose and macrogols. Side effects include gastrointestinal symptoms, like bloating, flatulence, vomiting and abdominal pain. These laxatives should not be used in patients with impaction. Lactulose should not be used in patients with galactosemia. Magnesium hydroxide should not be used in patients with hepatic and renal failure and patients with heart failure. Macrogols should not be used in patients with inflammatory bowel disease.

Stool softeners – These drugs soften stool by lubricating the rectum and anus. Examples are docusate, mineral oil and glycerin. They are suitable for patients with anal fissures and hemorrhoids. Side effects include abdominal cramps and nausea. These drugs should be used in patients with fecal impaction.

Antidiarrheals

Antimotility drugs – Antimotility drugs include opioids that stimulate the opioid receptors and cause constipation. Examples are loperamide and diphenoxylate.

Adsorbents – Adsorbents bind to bacterial toxins that irritate the gut mucosa and cause diarrhea. A good example is kaolin, which is formulated with pectin. Adsorbents can prevent the absorption of certain nutrients. Antidiarrheals should not be given to patients with bloody stools and features of sepsis.

Antimicrobials

Antibiotics

Those that inhibit the synthesis of cell walls

Penicillins – Penicillins inhibit the synthesis of cell walls by activating enzymes that autolyze the cell wall. They also inhibit crosslinking of peptidoglycan polymers used in making cell walls. Finally, they bind and antagonize enzymes used in the synthesis of cell walls (penicillin-binding proteins). Examples are narrow-spectrum drugs like penicillin G and penicillin V; very narrow-spectrum drugs like methicillin, oxacillin and nafcillin; wide-spectrum drugs that are penicillinase-susceptible (amoxicillin); ampicillin; ticarcillin; and piperacillin. Side effects include allergic reactions, such as rashes, fever, urticaria, hemolytic anemia, anaphylaxis, nephritis and joint swelling. Other effects are gastrointestinal symptoms like diarrhea and nausea.

Cephalosporins – Cephalosporins inhibit cell wall synthesis just like penicillins. They are, however, less susceptible to penicillinase released by MRSA. They include first-generation (cephalexin and cefazolin), second-generation (cefuroxime, cefaclor and cefprozil), third-generation (cefotaxime, ceftriaxone, ceftazidime and cefoperazone) and fourth-generation (cefepime and ceftaroline). Adverse effects include allergic reactions, like penicillins. Other effects include phlebitis and IM pain during injection.

Others
Others include aztreonam, carbapenems (meropenem, imipenem and doripenem) and beta-lactamase inhibitors (clavulanic acid and tazobactam). Side effects of aztreonam include gastrointestinal symptoms, headaches, vertigo and hepatotoxicity. Side effects of carbapenems include gastrointestinal symptoms and skin rashes. Symptoms of toxicity include encephalopathy, confusion and seizures.

Other drugs that act on the cell wall

These include vancomycin, fosfomycin, bacitracin, cycloserine and daptomycin. Side effects of vancomycin include nephrotoxicity, ototoxicity, fever and phlebitis. Rapid infusion can cause red man syndrome triggered by the release of histamine. Side effects of bacitracin include neurotoxicity, which manifests as tremors, psychosis and seizures. Side effects of daptomycin include myopathies.

Protein synthesis inhibitors

Mechanism of action – Protein synthesis inhibitors are bacteriostatic. They inhibit proteins used for synthesizing bacteria's ribosomes.

Examples – Tetracyclines (minocycline, tigecycline and doxycycline), macrolides (erythromycin, clarithromycin and azithromycin), chloramphenicol, clindamycin and oxazolidinones

Side effects

Tetracyclines – Gastrointestinal symptoms like nausea, diarrhea and enterocolitis, dysplasia and discoloration of tooth enamel, hepatic toxicity, ototoxicity, nephrotoxicity and photosensitivity

Macrolides – Skin rashes, GI distress, eosinophilia, hepatitis and inhibition of CYP450 enzymes that metabolize drugs like digoxin, carbamazepine and theophylline

Clindamycin – Includes GI distress, skin rashes, hepatitis, neutropenia and pseudomembranous colitis

Chloramphenicol – GI distress, bone marrow suppression, aplastic anemia, gray baby syndrome (cyanosis, anemia and heart failure) and inhibition of CYP450 enzymes that metabolize drugs, like warfarin, tolbutamide and phenytoin.

Aminoglycosides – Examples include gentamicin, kanamycin, tobramycin, neomycin and amikacin. Side effects include ototoxicity, nephrotoxicity and allergic skin reactions.

Antifolate drugs

Mechanism of action – Antifoloate drugs inhibit the synthesis of folic acids.

Examples – Sulfonamides (sulfisoxazole, sulfadoxine and sulfamethoxazole) and trimethoprim. Side effects of sulfonamides include hypersensitivity (Stevens-Johnson syndrome), polyarteritis nodosa, exfoliative dermatitis, rashes and fever. Other symptoms include GI distress, like diarrhea and vomiting; hepatitis; aplastic anemia; granulocytopenia; thrombocytopenia; nephrotoxicity; and competition with methotrexate and digoxin for the same binding site. Side effects of trimethoprim include leukopenia, megaloblastic anemia and granulocytopenia.

Fluoroquinolones – Fluoroquinolones interfere with the synthesis of DNA. Examples include first-generation drugs (norfloxacin), second-generation drugs (ofloxacin and ciprofloxacin), third-generation drugs (moxifloxacin, gemifloxacin and levofloxacin). Side effects include GI distress, insomnia, dizziness, rashes, headaches, phototoxicity, tendinitis and neurotoxicity. Also, they inhibit enzymes responsible for metabolizing theophylline and so increase their bioavailability.

Antimycobacterial drugs

Isoniazid – Isoniazid inhibits the synthesis of mycolic acid used in making the cell walls of mycobacterium. Side effects include insomnia, peripheral neuritis, restlessness and tremors. These symptoms are prevented by prescribing the drug with pyridoxine. Other side effects include hepatitis and hemolysis.

Rifampin – Rifampin inhibits the action of RNA polymerase. Side effects include orange staining of urine, sweat and tears. Other side effects include nephritis, hepatitis, rashes and thrombocytopenia. It also induces certain CYP450 enzymes and, therefore, quickens the elimination of a lot of drugs, including contraceptives, terbinafine, ketoconazole, anticonvulsants, methadone and warfarin.

Ethambutol – Ethambutol inhibits the synthesis of arabinosyltransferases responsible for synthesizing cell walls. Side effects include optic neuritis, reduced visual acuity and color blindness.

Pyrazinamide – Pyrazinamide's mechanism of action is unknown, but it has bacteriostatic properties. Side effects include arthralgia, hyperuricemia, GI distress, porphyria, hepatitis and photosensitivity.

Antifungals

Amphotericin B – Amphotericin B is a polyene that inhibits the permeability of fungi cells by binding to ergosterol. Side effects associated with its infusion include chills, fever, vomiting and hypotension. To prevent this from occurring, the drug should be infused slowly. Also, antipyretics, antihistamines and glucocorticoids should be given before the infusion. Other side effects include renal tubular acidosis, anemia and neurotoxicity.

Flucytosine – Flucytosine inhibits the synthesis of nucleic acids. Toxicity causes liver dysfunction, alopecia and bone marrow suppression.

Azoles – Azoles inhibit the synthesis of ergosterol and affect the cell membrane. Examples include ketoconazole, itraconazole, fluconazole and posaconazole. Side effects include vomiting, rashes, hepatotoxicity and diarrhea. Furthermore, ketoconazole inhibits the metabolism of warfarin, phenytoin oral hypoglycemics and cyclosporine. Ketoconazole increases the risk of infertility, gynecomastia and menstrual abnormalities.

Echinocandins – Echinocandins inhibit the synthesis of β(1-3)-glucan used for making the cell walls of fungi. Side effects associated with its infusion include fever, rashes, GI distress and flushing.

Griseofulvin – Griseofulvin inhibits the synthesis of nucleic acid and disrupts microtubular function. It is fungistatic. Side effects include headaches, GI distress, photosensitivity, confusion and elevated liver enzymes. It causes a disulfiram-like effect with alcohol and decreases the serum concentrations of warfarin.

Terbinafine – Terbinafine causes the accumulation of squalene, which disrupts the synthesis of ergosterol. It is fungicidal. Side effects include GI distress and rashes.

Antivirals

Drugs for herpes

Acyclovir – Side effects include headaches and GI distress. IV administration increases the risks for hypotension, seizures, delirium, nephrotoxicity and tremors.

Ganciclovir – Side effects include thrombocytopenia, granulocytopenia, seizures and elevated liver enzymes.

Cidofovir – Side effects include nephrotoxicity.

Foscarnet – Side effects include nephrotoxicity, neurotoxicity and ulceration of the genitourinary tracts.

Drugs for HIV

Nucleoside reverse transcriptase inhibitors (NRTIs)

Abacavir – Side effects include hypersensitivity reactions.

Didanosine – Side effects include pancreatitis, neurotoxicity, diarrhea, peripheral neuropathy and hyperuricemia.

Emtricitabine – Side effects include GI distress, asthenia, hyperpigmentation and headaches

Lamivudine – Side effects include headaches, insomnia and GI distress.

Tenofovir – Side effects include asthenia, GI distress, headaches and acute renal failure.

Zidovudine – Side effects include bone marrow suppression, thrombocytopenia, hepatitis, myalgia and insomnia. Azoles and protease inhibitors increase the bioavailability of this drug. Rifampin, on the other hand, decreases it.

Nonnucleoside reverse transcriptase inhibitors (NNRTIs)

Delavirdine – Side effects include teratogenicity, skin rashes and drug-drug interactions.

Efavirenz – Side effects include skin rashes, hypercholesterolemia and CNS toxicity.

Etravirine – Side effects include diarrhea, rashes and nausea.

Nevirapine – Side effects include rashes, hypersensitivity reactions like SJS and drug-drug interactions.

Protease inhibitors

Atazanavir – Side effects include peripheral neuropathy, GI distress, hyperbilirubinemia and rashes.

Darunavir – Side effects include rashes, GI distress and hepatitis.

Fosamprenavir – Side effects include paresthesias, rashes and GI distress.

Indinavir – Side effects include thrombocytopenia, hyperbilirubinemia, diarrhea and nausea.

Entry and fusion inhibitors

Maraviroc – Side effects include muscle and joint pain, cough, elevated liver enzymes and diarrhea.

Enfuvirtide – Side effects include hypersensitivity reactions.

Anti-influenza drugs

Amantadine and Rimantadine – Side effects include ataxia, dizziness, slurred speech and GI distress.

Oseltamivir and Zanamivir – Side effects include GI distress, cough and sore throat.

Drugs for viral hepatitis

IFN-α – Side effects include GI distress, neutropenia, alopecia, depression, myalgia, fatigue and thyroid dysfunction.

Adefovir Dipivoxil – Side effects include lactic acidosis, nephrotoxicity and hepatitis.

Entecavir – Side effects include nausea, headache, dizziness and fatigue.

Ribavirin – Side effects include hemolytic anemia and teratogenicity.

Antineoplastic Drugs

Alkylating agents

These drugs cause the breakage of DNA strands by alkylating the nucleophilic groups in the bases of DNA.

Cyclophosphamide – Side effects include GI distress, alopecia, myelosuppression, hemorrhagic cystitis, SIADH and pulmonary toxicity. IV hydration and premedication with mesna can reduce the risk of hemorrhagic cystitis.

Mechlorethamine – Side effects include alopecia, myelosuppression, GI distress and sterility.

Platinum analogs – This includes carboplatin, cisplatin and oxaliplatin. Side effects of cisplatin include hepatotoxicity, neurotoxicity, nephrotoxicity and GI distress. Side effects of carboplatin include myelosuppression, with a lesser risk of ototoxicity and nephrotoxicity.

Procarbazine – Side effects include myelosuppression, skin rashes and peripheral neuropathy.

Busulfan – Side effects include skin pigmentation, pulmonary fibrosis and adrenal insufficiency.

Dacarbazine – Side effects include GI distress, alopecia, myelosuppression, skin rashes and phototoxicity.

Antimetabolites

These drugs bind the synthesis of folic acid, pyrimidines and purines. They also suppress the immune response.

Methotrexate – Side effects include peripheral neuropathy, which can be prevented by taking the drug with folinic acid. Long-term use increases the risk of pulmonary fibrosis and hepatitis.

Mercaptopurine – Side effects include bone marrow suppression and hepatitis.

5-Fluorouracil (5-FU) – Side effects include myelosuppression, GI distress and alopecia.

Gemcitabine – Side effects include pulmonary toxicity and myelosuppression.

Natural products

Vinca alkaloids – These include vincristine, vinblastine and vinorelbine. They inhibit the formation of mitotic spindles. Side effects include GI distress, bone marrow suppression and alopecia. Vincristine has an increased risk of neurotoxicity and paralytic ileus.

Podophyllotoxins – These include teniposide and etoposide. They stimulate the breakage of DNA strands by blocking topoisomerase II. Side effects include GI distress and bone marrow suppression.

Camptothecins – These include irinotecan and topotecan. They damage DNA strands by blocking topoisomerase I. Side effects include diarrhea and myelosuppression.

Taxanes – Taxanes include docetaxel and paclitaxel. They block the formation of mitotic spindles. Side effects of paclitaxel include peripheral toxicity and hypersensitivity reactions. Side effects of docetaxel include bone marrow suppression and neurotoxicity.

Antibiotics

Anthracyclines – These include epirubicin, doxorubicin, daunorubicin and mitoxantrone. They block the action of topoisomerase II and cause the intercalation of DNA pairs. Side effects include cardiotoxicity, GI distress, severe alopecia and bone marrow suppression. Cardiotoxicity is particular to this group and includes heart failure, cardiomyopathy and arrhythmias.

Bleomycin – Side effects include pulmonary fibrosis, hypersensitivity reactions, alopecia, hyperkeratosis and blisters.

Mitomycin – Side effects include nephrotoxicity, hepatotoxicity, cardiotoxicity, pulmonary toxicity and severe bone marrow suppression.

<u>Others</u>

Tyrosine kinase inhibitors – Examples include imatinib, nilotinib and dasatinib. Side effects of imatinib include diarrhea, edema and CHF.

Inhibitors of growth factor receptors – Examples include trastuzumab, cetuximab and panitumumab. Side effects include vomiting, fevers, headaches and bone marrow suppression.

Rituximab – Side effects include myelosuppression and hypersensitivity reactions.

Interferons – Side effects include neurotoxicity and bone marrow suppression.

Asparaginase – Side effects include coagulopathy, acute pancreatitis and hypersensitivity reactions.

Proteasome inhibitors – Examples include carfilzomib and bortezomib. Side effects include heart failure, thrombocytopenia and hypotension.

<u>Hormonal agents</u>

Glucocorticoids – Side effects include hyperglycemia, fungal infections of the skin, cataracts, hypertension, skin atrophy, weight gain and brittle bones.

Gonadal hormone antagonist – An example is tamoxifen. Side effects of tamoxifen include vomiting, vaginal bleeding, hot flashes and venous thrombosis.

Gonadotropin-releasing hormone (GnRH) analogs – Examples include nafarelin and leuprolide. Side effects include gynecomastia, bone pain, hematuria, impotence and testicular atrophy.

Aromatase inhibitors – Examples include letrozole and anastrozole. Side effects include hot flashes, nausea, back pain, peripheral edema, diarrhea and dyspnea.

Chapter 4: Federal Requirements

This makes up 12.5% of the test content. Topic areas include:

Federal Requirements for Handling and Disposal of Nonhazardous, Hazardous, Pharmaceutical Substances and Waste

Classification of hazardous drugs

Hazardous drugs are classified based on these criteria:

1. The ability to trigger cancer in animals, humans or both (carcinogenicity)

2. The ability to trigger fetal defects and malformations (teratogenicity)

3. The ability to cause infertility or affect fertility

4. The ability to cause organ toxicity at small doses

5. The ability to trigger mutation of genetic materials (genotoxicity)

Hazardous drugs are grouped into biologic agents, immunosuppressive agents and antiviral drugs.

Product storage

Safety principles and protocols observed for the safe storage of hazardous drugs include:

1. Rotate inventory properly and regularly to reduce the risk of dispensing expired drugs.

2. Material Safety Data Sheets (MSDS) should be made available for all volatile chemical and oncology drugs. The MSDS lists protocols for first aid, cleaning up and handling hazardous drugs.

3. The inventory should be separated based on drug categories. This reduces the risk of errors during dispensing. Parenteral and oral drugs should be stored separately. Oncology drugs and volatile materials should be stored separately from others.

4. All hazardous drugs should be stored on shelves that are at or below eye level to allow proper visualization. They should have appropriate labels to alert the staff of their hazardous nature.

5. All staff should use the appropriate PPE when handling hazardous drugs.

6. Volatile substances should be stored in a cool environment with adequate ventilation to reduce the risk of fire explosions.

Product handling – When handling hazardous drugs, all personnel should wear the appropriate PPE that can protect for at least four hours if there is an accidental exposure.

Personal Protective Equipment (PPE)

Hair, head and shoe covers – These items of clothing should be worn to reduce contamination during compounding. They also protect workers from residues on the floors and other surfaces. Shoe covers should not be worn outside the compounding area to prevent cross-contamination.

Face and eye protection – The appropriate protection should be worn when handling hazardous drugs beyond the engineering control. Respirators with full facepieces can be used to protect the face and eyes. Safety glasses with side shields or eyeglasses are insufficient forms of protection because they do not protect from splashes.

Eye and face protection should be used when handling hazardous drugs beyond a C-PEC, when cleaning up spills or when working at or above the level of the eye. Eye goggles should be used with face shields to provide a wide and complete range of protection.

Respirators – Respirators are worn to protect the airways from airborne particles. They do not protect against vapors and gases and direct splashes. Masks do not provide protection and should not be worn for compounding or drug administration.

Gowns – Disposable gowns protect from splashes and spills of hazardous drugs. They also protect waste materials. Disposable gowns made with laminated materials, like polyethylene-coated polypropylene, provide better protection than gowns made of non-coated materials. Gowns should have no openings in the front and must not be closed from the back. Furthermore, they should be long sleeved, with closed elastic or knitted cuffs. They should be free from closures and seams that can allow drugs to slip through. Laboratory coats, isolation gowns, surgical scrubs and coverings made from absorbent materials are inappropriate coverings.

Gloves – Gloves should be ASTM-tested chemotherapy gloves. They should also be powder free. Gloves should be free from defects, weak spots and pinholes. Two pairs of gloves should be worn during disposing of hazardous materials, administration and compounding. Sterile preparations require sterile gloves.

Accidental exposure

Accidental exposure can occur during manufacturing, distribution, transportation, storage, receipt and administration of drugs. It can also occur during the handling of waste and repair of equipment. The MSDS should be consulted for accidental exposure. This sheet gives all the information on cleanup protocols, safe handling and first aid. All facilities storing hazardous drugs must have the appropriate first aid kits and eyewash. First aid should have PPEs, sodium hypochlorite, brushes, scoops, powders and warning signs for preventing movement to the contaminated area.

Proper waste disposal

Waste containers should be color coded, leakproof, labeled, spill-proof and made from nonreactive plastic. Used syringes, vials, tubings and contaminated PPEs can be discarded in yellow containers. Yellow containers should also be used to store expired or partially used hazardous drugs and contaminated items, like gowns, masks and booties.

Partially used vials, bags and syringes that are listed in the Resource Conservation and Recovery Act (RCRA) should be stored in black RCRA-coded containers. All hazardous wastes should be handled and transported by the appropriate personnel to the appropriate federally recognized facility.

OSHA

The Occupational Safety and Health Act (OSHA) was created in 1970 to enforce regulations and practices that will create a healthy and safe working environment for workers. Apart from enforcement, OSHA also works through outreach, sensitization, assistance and education programs. It is under the US Department of Labor and covers all work environments in both the private and public sectors. It also covers all jurisdictions under the US authority (Puerto Rico, the District of Columbia, American Samoa, the Virgin Islands, Wake Island, Guam, Johnston Island, Northern Mariana Islands and the Outer Continental Shelf Lands).

Employer responsibilities

Under the OSHA law, employers must:

1. Provide a working environment that is free from all forms of hazards. The environment must be compliant with all the standards and regulations set by OSHA.

2. Inspect the conditions of the work environment to be sure they are compliant with OSHA standards.

3. Provide the right equipment for employees and make sure the equipment is maintained properly.

4. Use the right color coding, labels, posters and signs to make employees aware of hazards.

5. Update all existing operating procedures and inform employees of the update.

6. Provide safety training manuals and literature written in a language employees understand.

7. Make sure that employees who handle chemical hazards are properly trained to do so. Training must include written manuals, safety data sheets and others.

8. Provide employees with the necessary training and medical check-ups.

9. Hang the OSHA poster in a visible area in the work environment.

10. Inform OSHA of all work-related injuries and deaths within eight hours of their occurrence. All work-related amputations and loss of vision must be reported within 24 hours.

11. Keep a written logbook and record of work-related injuries. This logbook must be accessible to employees and former employees.

13. Give all employees access to their medical and exposure records.

14. Not discriminate against employees for enforcing their OSHA rights.

15. Develop and use a health and safety program to reduce the incidence of work-related injuries.

Hazardous chemical materials

Hazardous chemical materials can be flammable, carcinogenic, poisonous, caustic or teratogenic. Employees are likely to be contaminated via ingestion, direct contact, inhalation, entry through broken skin or entry through the mucous membrane.

Hazard communication plan

This plan is used to inform employees of the different types of hazardous substances present in the work environment. Information is communicated via distinct warning labels on the substances. Employers must also provide an MSDS for the various hazardous chemicals available. These sheets are used to identify these chemicals based on their chemical names, trade names, manufacturers' names and addresses and the chemical family of the materials. They provide information on contact phone numbers for emergencies, physical data, and explain explosion data, fire and health hazards.

The National Fire Protection Association created a system for identifying hazardous materials. This system is made up of four diamond-shaped symbols. The red diamond at the top indicates a flammable material. The blue diamond on the left indicates that the material is hazardous to health. The white diamond at the bottom gives information on the type of hazard, including its radioactivity. The yellow diamond on the right describes the stability and reactivity of the material. This system also grades the severity of hazardous materials from zero to four, with zero meaning no hazard while four means extremely hazardous.

Exposure to radiation

CPhTs must avoid radiological exposure. This can be done by keeping personnel a good distance away from radiation sources, reducing contact time between personnel and radiation sources, labeling all radioactive materials and drugs, wearing the appropriate shields and monitoring the extent of radiation exposure.

Bloodborne Pathogens Standard

Blood-borne pathogens are infectious microbes present in the blood and other bodily fluids that can cause disease in affected workers. Examples include hepatitis, HIV, streptococcus, malaria, syphilis and others.

The Bloodborne Pathogens Standard was created by OSHA. It is a collection of precautions and safety protocols used by workers who are exposed to human blood and other potentially infectious materials; OPIM, such as semen, vaginal fluids, cerebrospinal fluids, peritoneal fluid, synovial fluid, saliva and amniotic fluids; any form of unfixed tissue/organ; HIV-containing cells and tissue cultures; organ cultures; and other tissues from experimental animals.

The principles of the Bloodborne Pathogens Standard include exposure control plans, universal precautions, hepatitis B vaccination, post-exposure follow-up, hazard communication and training, recordkeeping, engineering, workplace controls and use of PPE.

Universal precautions – Universal precautions were proposed by OSHA in 1992. These precautions are used for protecting all workers from blood-borne pathogens that may be transmitted via contact with infectious blood and bodily fluids from patients. Unlike standard precautions that are used for all bodily fluids, nonintact skin and mucous membranes, universal precautions are used for blood and OPIMs that are listed by OSHA.

Work practice controls – These are protocols used to reduce the risk of exposure to biohazards by altering the way tasks are performed. These principles include:

Use of appropriate handwashing procedures – This involves the use of handwashing sinks, running water, soap and paper towels. Hand sanitizers that contain at least 60% alcohol can be used for nonsoiled hands.

Appropriate disposal of sharps – Principles that can minimize needle picks include using sharps when there are no other alternate methods, disposing of used sharps quickly and appropriately and disposing of safety sharps immediately after use.

Appropriate handling of lab specimens – This involves observation of all standard precautions and transmission-based precautions in the collection and transportation of all laboratory specimens.

Appropriate handling of laundry – This involves the correct storage and transportation of soiled laundry that contains semisolid and liquid blood and OPIMs.

Appropriate cleaning of contaminated material – This includes appropriate cleaning of soiled surfaces before disinfecting with the appropriate disinfectant. It also includes appropriate cleaning and disinfection of contaminated laundry.

Engineering controls – These are devices that isolate or eliminate potential hazards from the workplace. Examples include handwashing, removal of hazardous materials and substituting them with safer options, such as substituting a corrosive chemical reagent with a safer one and using devices that can contain and isolate a hazard, like safety sharps, specimen containers, red bags and sharps disposal containers. Workplaces that are expected to use the OSHA standard include home care facilities, correctional institutes, research facilities and health-care facilities.

Fire safety and emergency plan

OSHA expects both employers and employees to be compliant with fire safety and emergency protocols. For example, there must be written procedures on what to do in case of a fire outbreak. These protocols must be routinely communicated to all members of staff. Fire exits must be marked, and fire extinguishers and pull boxes placed in strategic positions. The staff should be routinely trained, and the fire alarm and sprinklers routinely tested.

How to handle hazardous materials safely

1. To minimize the risk of exposure via inhalation, splashing and skin contact, hazardous drugs should be prepared in a vertical laminar flow hood.

2. The appropriate PPE should be worn (hypoallergenic gloves or nonpowdered latex gloves and disposable gloves).

3. Surfaces that have spills should be cleaned with alcohol. Handwashing should be strictly observed.

4. During disposal, toxic materials should be handled appropriately. In case of spills, the affected body part should be promptly washed with water. To preserve the integrity of the skin, it should not be scrubbed. In case of eye splashes, the eyes should be washed with water for about 15 minutes.

5. Contaminated personnel should be promptly taken to the emergency department.

Spills and cleanup

Pharmacies storing hazardous chemicals should have cleanup kits for spills. These kits should contain neutralizers and absorbents to clean alkalis, acids and other hazardous materials. Cleaning agents like bleach should be used for biological hazards.

Management of hazardous wastes

Hazardous wastes can be radioactive, toxic, ignitable, caustic, reactive or corrosive. They can also be in the form of sludges, gases, solids or liquids. They are classified into these categories:

F-list – Wastes from nonspecified sources
K-list – Wastes from specified sources
P-list/U-list – Wastes from commercial chemicals

Regulations for the management of hazardous waters also cover regulation of gaseous emissions, monitoring of groundwater, monitoring of waste disposal on land and storage of wastes in waste containers.

Waste containers for collecting hazardous wastes must be stored in the right containers. These containers must be properly labeled. Plastic containers are used for dressings, gloves, paper towels and soft waste materials. Rigid containers are used for collecting sharps. Waste containers should not be emptied by regular cleaning staff. They should only be emptied by the right personnel trained for doing so.

Federal Requirements for Controlled Substance Prescriptions

Controlled substances are drugs with a very high risk for abuse, addiction and dependency. These characteristics make their prescription highly regulated and monitored on both state and federal levels.

Schedules for controlled substances

These schedules for controlled substances are thoroughly discussed in chapter 2.

Prescriptions

Before a controlled substance can be prescribed, the following requirements must be met:

1. It must be prescribed by a clinician with a DEA license.
2. The pharmacist filling the prescription must have a license to dispense controlled substances.
3. Schedule I drugs like heroin cannot be prescribed or filled since they have no therapeutic effect recognized in the United States.
4. Schedule II drugs must be prescribed by a licensed clinician.
5. Schedule III, IV and V drugs can be prescribed by a clinician through a paper order, using the electronic prescribing of controlled substances (EPCS) or through a verbal order. Verbal orders are not accepted for Schedule II drugs.

At the pharmacy, the pharmacist can dispense controlled substances only if all the information is provided and verified:

1. The date of request of the drug
2. The patient's date of birth
3. The clinician's name, DEA number and address
4. The patient's name
5. The patient's address
6. The name of the drug
7. The strength of the drug
8. The dosage form
9. The number of refills
10. The directions for the use of the drug
11. The signature of the prescriber
12. The directions of use

Refills – The maximum number of refills for Schedule III, IV and V drugs is five. Only 90 pills can be allocated per time. Schedule II drugs can be used for only 30 days, and they have no refills.

Telephone orders and facsimiles

Prescription orders for Schedule III and IV drugs can be processed by fax or over the phone. Schedule II drugs cannot be processed in normal circumstances. Circumstances that can warrant a telephone order of a Schedule II drug include:

- When a practitioner prescribes the drug for compounding for direct administration (intraspinal infusion, IM, IV or other parenteral routes)
- When a practitioner prescribes the drug for patients living in long-term care facilities
- When a practitioner prescribes the drug for a patient in a hospice care program that is certified and/or covered by Medicare or a hospice care program with accreditation from the state

Oral orders for Schedule II drugs are allowed only in emergencies. The DEA defines an emergency as:

1. That which requires prompt administration of the controlled drug as a standard of care.
2. That in which the provision of a written prescription is not feasible.
3. That which warrants the practitioner to make a telephone order for the drug, provided the amount and dose are restricted to an amount used for treating the emergency. In this case, the practitioner must provide a written prescription to the pharmacy within a week of the telephone order. The pharmacist must inform the DEA if the written prescription is not received after seven days.

E-prescribing

Since 2010, practitioners have been allowed to transmit online prescriptions of Schedule II, III, IV and V drugs with SureScripts, the only certified software for doing so. Some states, however, still prohibit e-prescriptions for controlled substances.

Partial filling of prescriptions

The following conditions must be met for partial filling of prescriptions of Schedule II, III, IV and V drugs:

1. Record each partial filling in the same format as you would a refilling.
2. Do not dispense more than the total quantity of drugs prescribed.
3. Do not dispense six months from the date of the initial prescription for Schedule III and IV and 12 months for Schedule V.
4. Schedule II drugs can be dispensed partially if the pharmacist cannot provide the full quantity of an oral emergency or written prescription. However, the pharmacist must take note of the quantity supplied and supply the remainder within 72 hours.

Transferring prescriptions

The original prescriptions of Schedule III, IV and V drugs can be transferred for refilling between pharmacies, but this must be done only once. Pharmacies that share an electronic online database can transfer prescriptions as much as the refills order is allowed by the law and as initiated by the prescribing practitioner. However, prescriptions cannot be transferred for Schedule II controlled drugs.

Federal Requirements (FDA and DEA) for Controlled Substances

Ordering and transferring

The DEA Form 222 is used for ordering Schedule I and II substances. This form is available from the DEA free of charge and can be ordered online, via mail or by phone. Orders can be made only by licensed pharmacists. Schedules III, IV and V substances can be ordered directly from wholesalers or drug companies. When filling out the form, the pharmacist is required to fill in the date of order; the name of the company, including its address; the size of the drug packages per item; the number of packages; the DEA license number; and the signature. Only 10 different drug items can be ordered in a single form.

As the order is processed, the supplier is expected to fill in the DEA license number, the date of shipping of the packaging, the National Drug Code of each package and the indication of shipping. The supplier is expected to have a copy of the pharmacist's DEA certificate before processing the order.

Receiving and storing controlled substances

As soon as the drugs are received, the product name, package size, strength and quantity should be checked against the purchase order. Checking should be done by a pharmacist. Schedule II drugs should be checked against DEA Form 222. Schedule II drugs can either be stocked in a secured store or disbursed. The stock should be monitored continuously. Controlled substances may be stocked separately in a secure place or dispersed throughout the stock. Their stock must be continually monitored and documented.

Theft of controlled substances

As soon as a controlled substance is noted to be lost or stolen, the nearest DEA office must be promptly contacted and notified using DEA Form 106. The notification report must include the name of the company and its address, the date the item was lost or stolen, the pharmacist's DEA number, a list of all missing drugs and costs of purchase and an update from the local police. The pharmacist should keep the original copy of the report, while two copies are sent to the DEA. Some states will require that a copy be sent to the board of pharmacy. In some cases, a copy may be sent to the local police.

Damaged or outdated controlled substances

DEA Form 41 is used to report damaged and outdated controlled substances. The pharmacist must also attach a cover letter that describes the state of the drugs and request permission to destroy them. Retail pharmacies can make this request once a year. The request must be sent to the DEA at least two weeks before the scheduled date of destruction. This request must be approved before the drugs are destroyed. The process of destruction must be witnessed by at least two witnesses approved by the DEA.

Returning controlled substances

DEA Form 222 is used to return controlled substances. Returns can only be done by a licensed pharmacist. Returned substances must be labeled. The labels must contain the quantity of the drugs, product names, strengths and sizes. It must also contain the National Drug Code (NDC) numbers and the names of the manufacturers.

Recordkeeping

Pharmacists who store and dispense controlled substances must maintain a record for at least two years, although some states require that the record be kept for five years. Schedule II drugs must be recorded separately from other controlled substances. These records must be readily available for inspection by DEA officials.

Federal Requirements for Restricted Drug Programs and Related Medication Processing

Restricted drug programs

The FDA restricts access to certain medications because of the drugs' side effects and adverse effects. These drugs are managed through the Risk Evaluation and Mitigation Strategy initiative (REMS). When new drugs with certain side effects are produced, the FDA mandates companies to submit a REMS program that contains details on:

Communication plan – The drug manufacturers must educate all health-care workers and clinicians on the use of the drug, as well as how to safely use and prescribe the drug to patients.

Medication guide – This involves the creation of a well-written document that can be understood by patients and the public. The document should include safety information and risk warnings. This document must be given to the patients who are being prescribed the drug.

Elements to assure safe use – This is the use of systems to ensure that the drug is used appropriately.

Implementation system – The processes and principles of ensuring that the drug is used appropriately are described.

Timetable for submitting assessments – This is a timetable that describes how frequently the REMS program created by a drug company will be reviewed and assessed. FDA mandates that assessments be done one and a half years, three years and seven years after the drug is launched. Results of the assessment must be sent to the FDA.

Examples of drugs with significant restrictions include:

Thalidomide
This drug was originally manufactured for insomnia and sleep disorders. After it entered the European market, it was used off-label as an antiemetic for morning sickness. The drug, however, is teratogenic, causing birth defects in as high as 30% of infants. Thalidomide is used to treat multiple myeloma and erythema nodosum leprosum in the United States. Its availability is, however, controlled by the THALOMID REMS program. This program provides the drug to only certified members.

Clozapine
This is an atypical antipsychotic drug used to treat schizophrenics. It also has an off-label indication for bipolar disorder. Its side effects are severe and often life-threatening. They include CNS depression, agranulocytosis, seizures, hypotension, dementia, leukopenia, bone marrow suppression and myocarditis.

These side effects make the availability of this drug restricted to only registered members. Registered members are required to undergo serial monitoring of their absolute neutrophil count and white blood cell count. Members whose cell count falls below a certain cut-off are removed from the program and registered into the non–re-challengeable database. This database informs physicians and pharmacists or patients who are ineligible for clozapine.

Buprenorphine
This drug is used to treat opioid abuse disorder. The Drug Addiction Treatment Act (DATA) allows licensed physicians to prescribe buprenorphine for treating opioid addiction. Licensed physicians must have a valid registration number from

the DEA, a current state medical license and a specialty or subspecialty certification.

Isotretinoin

This drug is used to treat severe acne that is refractory to conventional treatment. The cut-off age is 12 years. This drug is teratogenic and can cause birth defects like visual and hearing impairments, mental retardation, facial dysmorphism and malformed or missing earlobes. To reduce the risk of these effects on the public, access to isotretinoin is restricted to registered members in iPLEDGE, a REMS program.

Phentermine and topiramate

These drugs are used to reduce appetite and restrict calorie intake. It is sold under the brand name Qsymia. These drugs are teratogenic, increasing the risks of clefting of the lips or palate. Access to these drugs is restricted by VIVUS, the manufacturer of the drug. Women of childbearing age are expected to use contraception during the use of this drug and confirm that they are not pregnant before they start the drug.

FDA Recall Requirements

Drug recalls are usually voluntary. In some cases, the FDA can put significant pressure on drug manufacturers to recall drugs that are deleterious to the public. Devices, supplements and medical supplies can also be recalled.

There are three types of drug recalls.

Class I – A drug with a high probability of causing adverse effects or death to the public is recalled.

Class II – A drug with a chance of causing reversible or temporary adverse effects, with a remote chance of causing adverse effects, to the public is recalled.

Class III – A drug that is unlikely to cause adverse effects to the public is recalled.

Steps involved in drug recalls

Step 1 – The adverse effect of the drug is reported to the FDA. The FDA can be notified in any of these ways:

- Directly by the manufacturers
- During an inspection of a manufacturing plant
- By the CDC
- Through various reporting channels

After notification, the FDA determines that the consistency and magnitude of notifications warrant a recall of the drug. The FDA informs the drug manufacturer.

Step 2 – The manufacturer consents to the recall. The manufacturer develops a strategy for recall and sends it for approval to the FDA. The strategy must be in-depth and extensive, and there must be a system for assessing the recall strategy.

Step 3 – Consumers are informed of the recall. Wholesalers and retailers are informed of the drug, including its size, product name, lot number, serial number or code and other information. They are also informed of the reason for the recall and steps on how to go about the process.

Step 4 – The recall is publicly announced in the weekly enforcement report.

Step 5 – The effectiveness of the strategy is checked. A recall strategy is said to be completed when all the corrected strategies are implemented and reviewed by the FDA. After the recall, the product is either reconditioned or destroyed. An investigation is then done to assess the cause of the defection.

Examples of inefficient drug recall in the United States include:

Fen-Phen (fenfluramine and phentermine) – This drug was manufactured by Wyeth-Ayerst Laboratories. It was indicated for weight loss via appetite suppression. It was recalled in 1997, 24 years after its release. Its adverse effects included pulmonary hypertension and valvular defects.

Diethylstilbestrol (DES) – This drug was produced by different manufacturers. It was indicated for preventing miscarriages. It was recalled in 1975, 37 years after its release. Adverse effects included teratomas in female fetuses.

Baycol – This is a brand name for cerivastatin, an HMG-CoA reductase inhibitor. It was manufactured by Bayer A.G. and recalled in 2001, four years after its release. Its adverse effects included rhabdomyolysis and AKI.

Vioxx – This is a brand name for rofecoxib, an NSAID. It was produced by Merck and recalled in 2004, five years after its release. Its adverse effect included increased risk for myocardial infarction.

Chapter 5: Patient Safety and Quality Assurance

This makes up 26.25% of test content. Topic areas include:

High-Alert/Risk Medications and Look-Alike/Soundalike (LASA) Medications

High-alert medications

These are medications with a very high risk for serious harmful effects if they are given erroneously. These drugs require caution in their prescription ordering, storage, administration and preparation. Other cautionary measures that should be observed include restricting access to these drugs, improving patient education on the use and side effects of these drugs, adding auxiliary labels, using automated alerts, performing double checks and more. These drugs can cause severe reactions like lethargy, delirium, bleeding, bradycardia, hypotension and hypoglycemia.

Drug categories

Adrenergic agonists – Norepinephrine, phenylephrine and epinephrine

Adrenergic antagonists – Propranolol, labetalol and metoprolol

Anesthetic drugs – Inhaled, general and IV (ketamine) and propofol

Antiarrhythmics – Amiodarone and lidocaine.

Antithrombotics – Direct thrombin inhibitors like argatroban and dabigatran; anticoagulants like unfractionated heparin; warfarin; low molecular weight heparin; thrombolytics like alteplase; factor Xa inhibitors like dabigatran, betrixaban, apixaban, rivaroxaban and edoxaban; and glycoprotein IIb/IIIa inhibitors like eptifibatide

Cardioplegic drugs – Chemotherapy agents and oral and parenteral hypertonic dextrose solutions greater than or equal to 20%

Solutions for dialysis

Intrathecal drugs – these drugs are injected into the spinal canal.

Inotropic drugs – Examples include milrinone and digoxin.

Insulin – Examples include IV and subcutaneous insulin.

Liposomal drugs – Examples include amphotericin B.

Sedatives – Examples include lorazepam and midazolam.

Opioids – This includes oral and parenteral forms.

Neuromuscular blocking drugs – Examples include vecuronium, succinylcholine and rocuronium

Sulfonylureas – Examples include tolbutamide, glyburide and glimepiride.

The Joint Commission on Accreditation of Healthcare Organizations has created a list of five high-alert medications that usually implicated. It also made a list of suggestions in reducing the risk of error during its use. These drugs are:

Insulin – Common risk factors for error include failure to check dose systems, keeping insulin and heparin vials side by side and mistaking U abbreviations for O, which can lead to administration of overdoses. Strategies for reducing these occurrences include implementing a check-and-balance system, where one nurse prepares the drug and another reviews it; separating insulin vials from heparin vials during storage; spelling out all units; and avoiding abbreviations.

Opiates – Common errors include confusing hydromorphone for morphine and patient errors (the rate of flow and concentration). Strategies for reducing these errors include educating clinical staff on the differences between hydromorphone and morphine and implementing checks and balances that prevent errors during patient administration.

Hypertonic sodium chloride – Errors include access to this hypertonic solution, making large quantities available and failure to implement checks and balances. Strategies for overcoming these errors include restricting access to this solution, standardizing the number of solutions available and using checks and balances for drug concentrations and pump rate.

IV heparin – Errors include storing heparin vials side by side with insulin vials, ambiguous labels and use of multidose containers. Strategies for eliminating these errors include storing heparin vials away from insulin vials, using standardized concentrations and using single-dose containers.

IV potassium chloride – Errors include easy access to this drug, mixing the drug extemporaneously and using unusual concentrations. Strategies for eliminating these errors include standardizing drug concentrations, restricting access to the drug and using commercially available premixes.

Look-alike/soundalike (LASA) medications

These are drugs that look alike in packaging or appearance or drugs that have similar spellings or pronunciations. Factors that increase the risk of error when handling LASA medications include illegible handwriting, similar packaging, ignorance of drug names, drugs with similar dosages and/or strengths, drugs with similar indications, drugs with similar frequency of dosing and ignorance of new drugs available in the pharmacy.

Strategies for reducing errors include:

1. Procurement

Reduce the number of drugs with multiple strengths.
As much as possible, avoid purchasing drugs with a similar appearance or packaging.

2. Storage

Differentiate labels of LASA drugs with tall man lettering. In tall man lettering, some parts of the names of the drugs are capitalized to differentiate soundalike drugs. In this case, the dissimilar letters are capitalized (rednisolo and rednisol, rednisolo and rednisolone).

Utilize extra warning labels for LASA drugs. The design of the warning labels should be consistent throughout the facility for easy recognition. For soundalike medication where tall man lettering cannot be used, brand or trade names should be added for differentiation. The nonproprietary name should be larger than the brand name. LASA drugs should be stored separately from the LASA pair if possible.

3. Prescribing

1. Use clear and legible writing on prescription forms.
2. The prescription forms should clearly state the name of the medication, including its dose, form and directions for use.
3. The patient's diagnosis should be added.
4. When ordering online, drug names should be written in tall man letters.
5. When placing orders over the phone, clearly pronounce the drug name and ask that the recipient of the call repeat the name.
6. Verbal orders should be used only for emergency calls if possible.

4. Dispensing/supply

Drugs should be identified only by their names and not by appearance or their location in the inventory. Before dispensing, check the dose and its appropriateness to the indication. Read all drug labels using the triangle check (checking the name of the drug against the prescription and label). Double-check during supply and dispensing.

5. Administration

Carefully perform the triangle check again before administering drugs. Educate people on the need to read and confirm the information on labels. Encourage staff to read back verbal orders for clarity and confirmation.

6. Monitoring

Pharmacies should monitor LASA drugs, update them and review them in the logbook.

7. Information

All relevant staff should have access to information on LASA drugs in the pharmacy.

8. Patient education

Patients should be informed of changes in the appearance of their medications. Educate patients on the need to inform their health-care providers on changes in the appearance of their drugs. Also encourage patients to learn the names of the drugs, including their brand and generic names.

Error Prevention Strategies

Tall man lettering – This term was coined by the Institute for Safe Medication Practices (ISMP) and is useful for reducing errors associated with LASA drugs. In this technique, the letters that differentiate one soundalike drug from the other are written in uppercase. For example, to differentiate prednisolone from prednisone, they are both written as rednisolo and rednisolone. The FDA advises drug manufacturers to use labels with tall man lettering to differentiate drugs. Furthermore, clinics, hospitals and health facilities are advised to use tall man lettering in their prescription order, drug labels, automated dispensing systems and admission records.

Separating inventory – This includes separating scheduled substances, hazardous drugs and high-alert medications from other inventories. It also includes separating LASA drugs.

Leading and trailing zeros – Leading zeros should be added before a decimal point. For example, ".5 mg" is wrong and should be written as "0.5 mg."

Trailing zeros must be avoided. For example, "5.0 mg" is wrong. It should be written as "5 mg." Inappropriate use of leading or trailing zeros can increase the risk of overdose, as much as 10 to 100 times the original dose.

Barcode usage – A barcode is a tool used to identify medications. This tool was created to ensure that the right drugs are given to the right patients in the right doses. Barcodes are electronic identifiers that reduce the risk of human error. They are printed on medications and are easily scannable to retrieve information, like the NDC number (used to identify the drug, the strength and dose), the batch number (which makes drug recalls easy) and the expiration date.

Electronic prescription record – This is used to reduce errors associated with dispensing drugs. It is an electronic record of data used to label drugs, dispense drugs and make payment requests. This tool is useful in preventing errors, like drug interactions, contraindications and duplicate prescriptions. Furthermore, electronic prescription records are used for drug utilization review and collaboration with prescribing clinicians.

Computerized Physician Order Entry (CPOE) – This is an electronic tool that allows prescribing clinicians to log in prescription orders. It reduces the risk of errors associated with illegible handwriting, harmful abbreviations and ambiguity.

Electronic DUR – This technology allows pharmacists to conduct drug utilization reviews online. This makes DURs proactive, comprehensive and timely.

Automated dispensing of medications – This tool reduces the risk of dispensing errors. It is used to perform tasks that are repetitive and tedious and that require a high level of concentration.

Procedures for internal quality control – This is used to evaluate workflow practices and analyze risks for error. For example, most dispensing systems use image recognition, alert systems and messaging to reduce the risk of errors when dispensing LASA drugs and high-alert drugs.

Limit the use of error-prone abbreviations – Some abbreviations can confuse because of their ambiguity or tendency for their meaning to be mistaken for another. The Joint Commission created a list of abbreviations that should not be used because of their high risk for errors. Examples include:

1. U – *Units* should be written instead.
2. IU – *International units* should be written instead.
3. QD – *Daily* should be written instead.
4. QOD – *Every other day* should be written instead.
5. QID – *Four times daily* should be written instead.
6. μg – *Micrograms* should be written instead.
7. SC/SQ – *Sublingual* should be written instead.
8. TIW – *Three times a week* should be written instead.
9. D/C – *Discontinue* should be written instead.
10. HS – *Half-strength* should be written instead.
11. cc – *Cubic centimeters* should be written instead.
12. AS/AU/AD – *Left ear/both ears/right ear* should be written instead.
13. OS/OU/OD – *Left eye/both eyes/right eye* should be written instead.
14. MSo4/MgSO4 – *Magnesium sulfate* should be written instead.
15. MS – *Morphine sulfate* should be written instead.

Issues That Require Pharmacist Intervention

Drug utilization review (DUR)

This is a structured process of reviewing the prescription, dispensing and use of drugs. It is an ongoing process that is authorized by legal entities. Another name for drug utilization review is medication utilization evaluation. Drug utilization review is useful in reducing the cost of purchasing drugs. This is especially true for countries where the aging population lives longer due to improved health systems and increasingly depends on drugs to manage chronic diseases.

Types of drug utilization review

Prospective review – This review is done before drugs are dispensed to patients. In this stage, the pharmacist assesses the patient's drug history and makes note of issues that can affect the patient's compliance and adherence. For example, pharmacists usually assess the dose of medications, the route of administration, side effects and interactions with food, herbal supplements and other drugs. When prospect review is done as a component of an online claims process, computerized algorithms are used for efficiency.

Drug issues that are readily identified by a prospective review include:

1. Drug abuse
2. Disease contraindications to drugs
3. Modification of drug dosage
4. Drug-drug interactions
5. Patient precautions (often identified via patient history)
6. Substitution of formulas
7. Inappropriate duration of therapy

Concurrent review – The review is done during the commencement of treatment. It involves continuous monitoring of medication therapy to improve the patient's outcome. Pharmacists can observe the patient's response and quickly intervene if there are side effects and inform the prescribing clinician of these side effects. Due to the integrated use of electronic prescribing, prescribers can do a concurrent review during prescription. This makes it easier for the pharmacist to intervene when necessary. Concurrent review is used to monitor these issues:

1. Drug-drug interaction
2. Drug-disease interaction
3. Patient precautions (gender, age and others)
4. Overutilization of drugs
5. Underutilization of drugs
6. Modification of dosages
7. Therapeutic interchange and substitution

A good place to see concurrent review in action is in inpatient facilities, where patients are typically treated with multiple drugs. Concurrent review can help the clinicians quickly identify duplicate therapy, drug-drug interactions, inappropriate duration of therapy and more.

Retrospective review – This review is done after the patient has received the drug. This review aims to detect challenges with the prescription, dispensing and administration of medications, and to develop strategies to prevent such challenges from recurring. Retrospective review is used to identify these challenges:

1. Clinical abuse
2. Drug-drug interactions
3. Incorrect dosage of drugs
4. Underutilization of drugs
5. Overutilization of drugs
6. Inappropriate duration of therapy
7. Substitution of formulas
8. Inappropriate use of generic drugs
9. Disease contraindications to drugs

Steps in drug evaluation

1. Identify optimal use – The organization creates a set of criteria for assessing optimal use of drugs. These criteria are usually outcome-focused (focused on therapeutic outcomes).

2. Evaluate actual drug use – The actual use of drugs is evaluated. The data obtained is then compared with that of optimal use. This step requires the implementation of algorithms to identify eligible subjects for obtaining data.

3. Evaluation – An algorithm is used to identify eligible subjects. The data obtained from them are then compared with that of optimal use. In this process, the algorithm detects discrepancies between the two sets of data.

4. Intervention – The results of the comparison are interpreted, and action plans are created and aimed at the areas of concern.

5. Evaluation of the review program – The effectiveness of the drug review program is evaluated. This step is necessary to improve the efficiency of future reviews.

6. Report the findings of the review program – The findings from the evaluation of the review program are communicated to the appropriate unit.

Adverse drug event (ADE)

Adverse drug events are unpleasant, unwanted and harmful reactions that are caused by drug interventions.

Classification of adverse drug events

Type A reaction – This is also known as an augmented reaction. This reaction is dose dependent and typically predictable.

Type B reaction – This is also called a bizarre reaction. It is unpredictable and idiosyncratic. It is not dose dependent.

How to prevent adverse drug reactions

Identify susceptible patients – This involves the collection of detailed patient history to recognize patients who are at risk. During the history-taking, important data—like the patient's age, ethnicity, pregnancy status and gender—can help screen at-risk patients. Another aspect of history-taking is asking for a detailed drug history to rule out or confirm prior adverse reactions.

Treatment plan – This involves the creation of safe treatment plans that take into consideration the adverse effects of the prescribed drugs. For example, a patient who has been prescribed methotrexate will benefit from a prescription of folic acid to mitigate the effects of folate deficiency. Another example is placing patients on diuretics on serial renal function monitoring.

Pharmacovigilance – This is the practice of collecting data for the early detection of adverse effects. It also includes patient monitoring and assessment and the use of prevention strategies. In pharmacovigilance, information is obtained not only from patients but also from health workers and medical literature. Data is usually obtained from the drug company, analyzed and interpreted and then reported to the drug regulatory agency.

Over-the-counter (OTC) recommendation

OTCs are drugs that do not require a prescription for their procurement. Recommendation of OTCs should be made only by a pharmacist, not a CPhT.

Before a pharmacist recommends an OTC, a history of the patient's illness must be collected. Nonspecific symptoms—like fever, headaches and congestion—can be managed with OTC drugs. As the pharmacist obtains the history, he or she must rule out serious symptoms or chronic mild symptoms. For example, persistent headache may be a sign of cardiovascular disease, and chronic fever can point to a chronic inflammatory response that needs clinical management. After obtaining a history of the patient's complaints, the next step is to obtain a medical history and drug history. The medical history aims to identify diseases that are incompatible with certain OTCs.

For example, a patient with hypertension will not benefit from certain anticongestants with vasoconstrictor properties. The drug history is necessary to rule out or confirm drug allergies and adverse effects and eliminate the risk of drug-drug reactions. Finally, the pharmacist should obtain a history of the medications the patient has taken so far and the patient's desire for specific medications.

Before dispensing the drug, the pharmacist should educate the patient on the drug's mechanism of action, dosage, indications, contraindications and side effects. There are some factors the pharmacist should keep in mind to promote compliance. For example, most patients prefer drugs with shorter frequencies of dosing (once-a-day doses are easier to follow compared to twice-a-day or three-times-a-day doses).

Therapeutic substitution

This is the process of replacing a drug with another drug from the same class that has the same clinical effect as the substituted drug. Therapeutic substitution is done only by a pharmacist and not a CPhT. Pharmacists can decide to substitute a drug to save cost, prevent adverse effects or provide a substitute when the initial drug is unavailable. A pharmacist may or may not inform the prescribing clinician of the substitution. The decision to inform depends on state laws, the patient's medical condition and the type of drugs involved.

Because of the risks involved with therapeutic substitution, most clinicians do not approve of it. Furthermore, some drugs should not be substituted without informing the prescribing clinician. Some of these drugs include antiseizure drugs, antihypertensives and antidepressants. Pharmacists can substitute a drug without identifying the patient. To prevent this from happening, the prescribing clinician should write "DAW," "May not substitute" or "Do not substitute" on the prescription note.

The following principles should be observed to encourage efficient therapeutic substitution:

Competence of the pharmacist – The pharmacist should be competent and able to provide service according to the standards of care. This means that the pharmacist should have the required skills and knowledge of the drug being dispensed and the patient's condition.

Appropriateness of information – The pharmacist has the right level of information required to make a substitution that is both safe and effective for the patient.

Prescription – The pharmacist has an appropriate, current and authentic prescription.

Appropriate adaptation – The pharmacist can adapt the prescription to the patient's needs and condition.

Informed consent – The pharmacist must inform the patient before making any substitution to the prescription.

Documentation – The pharmacist must document any substitution made, including the reason for doing so and any follow-up plan.

Notify the prescribing clinician – The pharmacist must inform the prescribing clinician of the substitution. This information must be given no later than 24 hours after the event.

Misuse

This is the act of using a drug/substance for a nonindicated purpose. *Substance use disorder* describes an abnormal set of behaviors whereby affected patients use psychoactive substances even when experiencing problems due to using. These problems can be physical or psychological. The term *substance use disorder* has a less negative connotation than *substance addiction*, *substance abuse* and *dependence*.

Addiction is the tendency to keep taking psychoactive drugs even in the face of physical and psychological complications. The risk for addiction depends on the drug's route of administration, the drug's ability to induce withdrawal symptoms or tolerance, the drug's time of onset and the rate at which the drug crosses the blood-brain barrier. Drugs that are commonly abused include illegal drugs, like club drugs, anabolic steroids, inhalants, cocaine, marijuana, heroin and methamphetamine. Also, prescription drugs can be abused.

Commonly abused prescription drugs include opioids, anxiolytics and sedatives. Patients abuse prescription drugs by using someone else's prescription drugs, taking more doses than prescribed, administering a drug in a different way than intended (crushing and snorting them instead of swallowing them as prescribed). Another way of misusing drugs is pretending to have a medical condition to obtain a prescription or an OTC drug.

Factors that increase the risk for drug misuse include biological factors, such as mental illness, a genetic predisposition for addictive behavior and gender (men have a twofold increase of abusing drugs than women). Environmental factors, such as impoverished communities, communities with access to drugs and poor neighborhoods, are also implicated. Other factors include the use of drugs from an early age, antisocial behavior, aggressive behavior, poor parenting, poor mechanisms to cope with stress, long work hours, history of drug abuse in parents or siblings, parental divorce and sensation-seeking behavior.

Pharmacists' interventions in drug misuse include inspecting prescriptions for alterations and falsifications and alerting other pharmacies of such prescriptions. Furthermore, pharmacists can collaborate with prescribing clinicians to track the prescription and dispensing of opioids to patients.

Withdrawal syndromes

Opioid

Symptoms are usually not fatal. Symptoms are anxiety, tachypnea, diaphoresis, lacrimation, yawning, rhinorrhea, diarrhea, anorexia, tremors, fever, tachycardia, hypertension and stomach cramps.

Alcohol

Alcoholic withdrawal symptoms are fatal. Mild symptoms include headaches, tremors, weakness, diaphoresis, tachycardia, hypertension, seizures, gastrointestinal symptoms and hyperreflexia. Symptoms progress to involve alcoholic hallucinosis characterized by visual and auditory hallucinations and nightmares. Delirium tremens is a late-onset symptom characterized by increasing anxiety, depression, sweating, disorientation, autonomic features, altered personality, tachycardia and hyperthermia.

Anxiolytic

Withdrawal symptoms of benzodiazepines are not life-threatening. However, withdrawal from barbiturates can mimic life-threatening symptoms similar to delirium tremens. Features of benzodiazepine withdrawal are tachycardia, tachypnea, hyperpyrexia and seizures. Features of barbiturate withdrawal include restlessness, increasing anxiety, hyperreflexia, muscle weakness, delirium, seizures that can progress to status epilepticus, insomnia, visual and auditory hallucinations and death.

Nicotine

Nicotine causes strong physical dependence. Features are irritability, difficulty concentrating, anxiety, depression, insomnia, hunger, GI disturbances, headaches and weight gain.

Cannabis

Withdrawal symptoms of cannabis are generally mild because they do not produce profound physical dependence. Dependence is more psychological. Features include insomnia, nausea, irritability, anorexia and depression.

Adherence

Drug adherence is a patient's ability to follow through with a drug regimen. Adherence to care regimens becomes problematic for patients with chronic diseases.

Factors that affect adherence include:

Patient factors – This includes the age of the patient (children and elderly patients are least likely to adhere to drug regimens), concerns about a drug's adverse effects, forgetfulness, apathy and indifference, reduction in the severity of symptoms, mix-up of the dose's prescription and physical difficulties in taking a drug.

Drug factors – Adverse effects, frequent dosing, polypharmacy, unpleasant smell or taste of the drugs.

Factors that can improve adherence include:

Simplifying the drug regimen – A common strategy to improve adherence is simplifying the drug regimen. For example, using once-a-day drug dosages greatly increases the patient's chances of adhering to the drug regimen. Another tactic is to synchronize drug dosing with the patient's activities, such as taking drugs before a meal or just before going to bed. Adherence is a cause for concern in elderly patients because of factors like polypharmacy, decreased cognition and lack of supervision.

Education – Patients' understanding of their conditions improves adherence. Studies have shown that patients who understand their conditions and the impact of their drug regimens are twice as likely to follow through with their treatment plans. Health-care providers can improve adherence by using simple, conventional language, involving the patients' caregivers and dividing the education into short blocks.

Eliminating bias – It is necessary to identify and remove bias that affects adherence. In this case, patient education is a useful tool in addressing the patients' intentions, beliefs and self-efficacy.

Patient communication – This includes not only pharmacist-patient communication but communication with other members of the health team. The pharmacist-patient communication channel is a challenging one because most patients do not understand what is being communicated about their health condition. This phenomenon is fueled by poor communication techniques used by health workers and the inability of health-care providers to interpret both verbal and nonverbal cues.

Post-immunization follow-up

A primary reason for post-immunization follow-up is to follow up with patients with adverse effects after immunization (AEFI). These adverse effects can range from mild to severe reactions. These reactions can be classified into:

Vaccine product–related reaction – This reaction is caused by the properties inside the vaccine. For example, some patients can experience edema of the limbs after a DTP vaccine.

Vaccine quality defect–related reaction – This reaction is caused by a defect in a vaccine and the device for administering it. For example, if the manufacturer does not inactivate the poliovirus in a vaccine, it can cause paralytic polio.

Immunization error–related reactions – These are reactions caused by inappropriate handling, prescription and administration of vaccines. This reaction is preventable. A good example is when a vaccine is administered from a contaminated vial.

Immunization anxiety–related reaction – This reaction is triggered when a patient is anxious about receiving a vaccine.

Coincidental event – This reaction is caused by another factor apart from errors with immunization, the vaccine or immunization anxiety. For example, a patient experiences fever after receiving a vaccine, but the fever is caused by malaria.

Serious events – These are AEFI reactions that are life-threatening, cause death, require extensive inpatient admission, cause disability, manifest as a birth defect/congenital anomaly or require urgent medical intervention.

Event Reporting Procedures

Medication errors

The National Coordinating Council for Medication Error Reporting and Prevention (NCCMERP) in the United States defines medication errors as a preventable occurrence that can cause an inappropriate use of a medication or patient harm when the drug is still under the administration of a health-care provider, a consumer or a patient.

Medication errors can be classified into administration errors, monitoring errors, prescribing errors, dispensing errors and transcription errors. The following are steps involved in reporting medication errors:

1. As soon as a health worker notices a medication error, the Medication Error Report must be quickly filled out. The details to be completed include the patient's name, the details of the prescription, the hospital number, the details of the error, including the type of error, the name of the medicine given and the dose.
2. This form should then be forwarded to the pharmacy department within 24 hours.
3. The medication safety officer is responsible for assessing the severity of the incident and performing a root cause analysis. The person is also responsible for making a report to the Medication Safety Committee. The medication safety officer should review the error and take measures to prevent a future recurrence.

Generally, systems for reporting medication errors include:

Voluntary reporting – Health-care providers report errors without any obligation or compulsion to do so.

Open reporting – Health-care workers of any status can make a report of a medication error.

Anonymous reporting – The health-care provider makes a report without identification.

Stand-alone reporting – Reports on medication errors are stored in a database that is accessible only by the members of the review team.

Paper and electronic-based database reporting – Medication errors can be reported via either an electronic means or pen and paper.

Adverse effects and product integrity

In the United States, the FDA has the adverse event reporting system (FAERS) and the Vaccine Adverse Event Reporting System (VAERS). Created in 1969, the AERS is a computerized safety surveillance system for monitoring medication errors and adverse effects of therapeutic biologic products and drugs. Reporting is voluntary and can be done by health-care providers, consumers and patients.

To make a report, patients are expected to fill in the following information: the age, weight and gender of the affected patient; the type of event; the date of its occurrence; the outcome from the event; the name of the product; the name of the manufacturer; the date of use of the product; the diagnosis/indication for use; a detailed description of the event and biodata of the person filling in the report.

Reports can be made online, via mail or by telephone. The reports are then reviewed by a team of experts. If there is a cause for concern, further studies are done. The FDA then takes action to protect public health and improve the product's safety. Some of the actions taken include restricting the drug's use, performing a recall or providing safety information or guides about the product.

There are limitations involved in the use of the data provided to AERS. For example, because the FDA does not require that a causal relationship be established between the event and the implicated product, most reports do not contain enough information for a thorough evaluation.

MedWatch

Created in 1993, MedWatch is a part of the AERS run by the FDA. It is used to report sentinel events and adverse events. Reporting systems are voluntary and can be done by both health-care providers and users. The data provided to MedWatch is available to the public. Apart from surveillance, MedWatch is also involved in drug recalls and safety education and communication.

To make reports, patients, consumers and health-care providers use the one-page form for reporting. Reporting can be done online or by fax, mail or telephone. If MedWatch detects a hazard signal for a medical product, the FDA alerts the public by making a recall or withdrawal or announcing changes to medical labels or product guides. Information is disseminated via the MedWatch website.

Alerts are made only on products approved by the FDA. These products include prescription and OTC drugs; medical devices like pacemakers, breast pumps and hearing aids; biologics like gene therapies and blood derivatives; combination products like nasal sprays and metered-dose inhalers; cosmetics; food; nutritional products like supplements and infant formulas; vaccines; tobacco products; drugs for animals; pet food and pet devices.

Near miss

A near miss is a medication error that is detected before it gets to the patient. These errors are detected either by chance or through systemic designs that have been put in place. The AHRQ, however, describes a near miss as a medication error that was disrupted by chance.

Root-cause analysis (RCA)

This is the process of discovering the cause of problems. It involves the use of techniques, tools and approaches for analyzing cause and effect. RCA is grouped under total quality management. It works in tandem with quality improvement.

In pharmacy, an RCA is used to identify the causes of sentinel and adverse effects. It is also focused on assessing processes and systems and not individuals.

Features of a successful RCA

1. It should be able to identify the processes and systems required to reduce the recurrence of adverse/sentinel events and improve performance.
2. It should be focused on the performance of systems and systems and not on individual performance.
3. It should give a comprehensive understanding of the events being investigated so that it can address the root of the problems.
4. It should actively involve leaders in problem-solving, decision-making and implementation.
5. It should actively involve members who are impacted by the problem or involved in the processes being reviewed.
6. It should be consistent.
7. Methods used should reflect current standards of practice and research literature.

How to do an RCA

Create a team – A team is created to assess the processes and systems that led to the event. The team ideally consists of:

1. Leaders – These are people involved in administrative duties who can create policies that can bring about change.
2. Frontline workers – These are people directly involved in the processes/systems that led to the event.
3. RCA experts – These are people who know how to use RCA in creating change.
4. Others – These are individuals who are directly involved in the event or know about the event.

Create a problem statement – The team describes the event clearly and concisely. The problem statement should be chronological. Information about the event can be gathered by:

1. Reviewing the documents involved (compounding log, prescription orders, counseling log and electronic entries)

2. Evaluating the environment where the event took place
3. Assessing the packaging and labeling of the drugs
4. Interviewing staff who witnessed or were directly involved in the event

Generate a flowchart – A flowchart is created to visualize the timeline of events. To analyze all the root causes of the event, in this stage it is important to ask why. Unanswered questions should warrant more research and data collection.

Identify root causes – The team evaluates the root cause by using comments and feedback from team members to differentiate the root cause from contributing factors.

Make a statement of the report – The team creates a statement describing the relationship between the cause of the problem and its effects. Care must be taken to ensure that it was the processes and systems that were critically assessed, not individuals.

Create an action plan – Strategies to prevent or reduce the incidence of risk are created after brainstorming within the team. Action plans should be created for each root cause. Doing so, however, depends on the quantity and quality of resources available.

Establish the measures of assessment – A set of criteria is created for evaluating the effectiveness of the action plan.

Communicate – The results of the RCA are communicated to the members of the organization.

Types of Prescription Errors

Types of errors

Prescribing errors – These errors occur when prescription orders are written. It can be caused by illegible handwriting, human factors, ignorance of drugs, rule violations, use of dangerous abbreviations and insufficient patient information.

Prescribing errors can be made by pharmacists, physician assistants, nurses, physicians and any clinical practitioner with the legal ability to prescribe drugs.

Dispensing errors – These errors are caused by CPhTs and pharmacists. They include drug contamination, prescription of wrong drugs, wrong dosages, wrong drug forms, wrong drug strength, the erroneous constitution of drugs and others. To reduce the risk of this type of error, the CPhT should have a good knowledge of dosage calculations, generic and trade names of drugs, drug pharmacology, pharmacokinetics and pharmacodynamics and LASA drugs and principles.

Administration errors – These errors occur when a drug is administered. Risk factors include environmental and human errors.

Forms of errors

Wrong drug – The wrong medication is given. To prevent this from occurring, the prescription order must be confirmed. This can be done by confirming the information on the drug label after it is brought out of the store, before removing it from the container and before administration. The expiration date should also be confirmed.

Wrong dose – An inappropriate drug dose is given (underdose or overdose). To prevent this from occurring, the CPhT should be skilled in calculating drug doses. Furthermore, the appropriate unit-dose systems should be used.

Wrong patient – A drug is given to another patient with no indication for the drug. To prevent this from occurring, the patient's name and other identifiers must be confirmed. Before administering the drug, the patient should be informed about the name of the drug, including its action, precautions, dosage and side effects.

Wrong time – To prevent administering a drug at the wrong time, the correct time should be confirmed on the prescription order or drug chart.

Wrong route – This can be avoided by confirming the route of administration on the patient's drug chart. In case of doubts, confirmation should be obtained from the prescribing clinician.

Wrong technique – This can cause undermedication or overmedication. To prevent this from happening, the physician should be familiar with the appropriate techniques.

Wrong information on the patient's chart – This error can cause all sorts of prescription and administration errors. To prevent this from happening, the date and time of administration of drugs should be accurately recorded. Furthermore, the patient's reactions to the drug—which may include side effects, allergies and adverse effects—should all be included.

Risk factors for errors

Human factors – This includes lack of recall, distractions, inability to notice details, failure to follow the standards of practice, malpractice and negligence. Some factors that contribute to human error include:

Fatigue – Fatigue can make workers distracted, impatient and unable to pay attention. It also increases the risk of delayed reaction, inaccuracy, memory lapses, irritability and reduced enthusiasm and empathy. Because health workers typically work long hours in health facilities, the risk for fatigue is extremely high. Long work hours and shift rotations that can affect the sleep cycle increase the risk of stress and fatigue. As a rule of thumb, health workers should not work more than 12 hours a day and 60 hours a week.

To reduce the incidence of fatigue in a work environment, health workers, including their employers, should be educated on the effects of fatigue and the benefits of rest and sleep. Strategies to relieve fatigue during work hours should be implemented. Some of these strategies include scheduled naps, efficient work schedules and rotations, the use of ambient light for night-shift workers and the use of technology like infusion pumps and barcoding.

Noise – This includes both external and internal noise. Noise can disrupt attention and focus and increase the risk for errors.

Poor lighting – Adequate lighting improves visibility and reduces the risk for errors. Poor lighting can cause workers to misread labels, including dosages and names.

Poor management – It is important to supervise and manage staff to reduce the risk of errors. CPhTs should be supervised by pharmacists at all times. Another aspect of management is seeing to it that the staff's welfare needs are met. Some of these needs include efficient rotation and scheduling, provision of AC, proper lighting, elimination of noise, implementation of safety protocols and more.

Illegible handwriting – This is the second most common cause of errors. Illegible writing makes it hard to confirm prescriptions and can increase the time it takes for a patient to start therapy. It is important for prescribing clinicians to use clear writing. They can dictate the prescription or write them with an electronic tool.

Insufficient monitoring of the patient – The patient should be monitored before and after a drug is administered. This is especially true for high-alert drugs. For example, before administering an analgesic, a pain scale should be used to grade the patient's perception of pain. Another method for monitoring a patient's response to drug therapy is through diagnostic blood and radiological tests. Tests like INR, clotting time, complete blood count, urine m/c/s, chest x-ray and serum glucose are used to monitor a patient's response to therapy. Drugs with a narrow therapeutic index require serial monitoring to detect the onset of adverse effects. For example, patients on lithium-ion for bipolar disorders require serial monitoring of white blood cell count and thyroid.

Insufficient drug knowledge – Some patients do not know much or anything at all about their medications. Such patients are at risk of abusing their drugs either by underdosing or overdosing. Patients should be taught about their medications and encouraged to ask questions, including about a drug's mechanism of action, indications, contraindications and side effects.

Insufficient patient information – This includes identifying information, like the patient's sex, age, allergies, height, lab test value, vital signs, diagnosis and ability to pay for the medications. Insufficient patient information increases the risk for adverse effects and drug interactions.

Rule violations – When standards of practice are violated, the risk for errors increases greatly.

Hygiene and Cleaning Standards

Handwashing – Handwashing can reduce the transmission of infectious diseases of the respiratory and digestive systems by as much as 50%. Hand hygiene should be observed before and after contact with a patient, immediately after handling bodily fluids, after touching nonintact skin and mucous membranes, immediately after removing gloves, before moving from a contaminated to a decontaminated area, after coming in contact with a patient's environment, after using medical equipment, after using the restroom, before eating and after coughing or sneezing.

Tips for effective handwashing

1. Use liquid soap instead of bar soaps. Liquid soaps stored in jars with nozzles are easier and less messy than bar soap.
2. Use running tap water instead of water basins.
3. Use paper towels instead of cloth towels.
4. Put up pictures of handwashing techniques close to the sinks.
5. Wet your hands with clean, running water.
6. Lather your hands by rubbing them with soap, including the backs of your hands, between your fingers and under your nails.
7. Scrub your hands for at least 20 seconds.
8. Rinse your hands well under clean, running water.
9. Dry your hands using a paper towel.
10. Hand sanitizers that contain at least 60% alcohol can be used in place of soap and water if the hands are not dirty.

Personal protective equipment – This is extensively covered in chapter 4.

Cleaning of countertops, counting trays and equipment – Clean counting trays with isopropyl alcohol after each use. A different tray should be used for hazardous drugs, like chemotherapy agents.

When using laminar flow hoods, the appropriate PPE should be worn. Furthermore, the technician should remove all jewelry, watches and cosmetics before using the hood. Headgear should be worn to prevent contamination.

Chapter 6: Order Entry and Processing

This makes up 21.25% of test content. Topic areas include:

Procedures for Compounding Nonsterile Products

Suspensions

Suspensions are liquid formulations that have solid particles suspended in a liquid. Although it is easy to compound suspensions, keeping them stable is challenging. To compound suspensions, the powder is first ground into fine particles in a process called trituration. Thereafter, a small amount of liquid is added to the powder in a process called levigation. This process is done slowly and steadily, all the while mixing the solution consistently until a paste is formed.

A suspending agent is added to the mixture in a high-speed mixer before it is dispersed. Finally, the dispersed mixture is stored in a bottle that is protected from light. Suspensions should have clear labels that encourage the user to shake well before use.

Solutions

Unlike suspensions, a solution does not require shaking before it is used. Solutions can be sterile or nonsterile. Sterile solutions include ophthalmic solutions and parenteral solutions. Nonsterile solutions include topical solution, otic solution and oral solution. Before a solution is compounded, it is important to confirm the solubility of the active ingredients. It is also important to compound solutions slowly.

Elixirs

These are oral drug formulations that contain alcohol and syrup. To compound elixirs, alcohol-soluble ingredients are dissolved in alcohol, while water-soluble ingredients are dissolved in water. The two solutions are then mixed. For successful compounding, the alcohol should be concentrated. During compounding, the mixture should be continuously stirred.

Emulsions

This is a form of suspension made with an emulsifier and two types of liquids. Water-in-oil emulsions are very greasy and suitable only for external use. Oil-in-water emulsions, on the other hand, are used orally and are not greasy. The two methods for creating emulsions are the continental/dry gum method and the English/wet gum method.

The dry gum method is preferred. In this method, gum acacia is mixed in oil. Water is added to the mixture before it is then triturated to the appropriate color and consistency. In the wet gum method, water and gum acacia are mixed, and then the oil is added to the mixture.

Ointments

These are oil-based semisolid drug formulations. Powders or crystals, like salicylic acid and hydrocortisone, are compounded into ointments or creams. Mixing is done either on a slab or in a mortar. Liquids are added gradually, and the mixture is stirred continuously. Insoluble powders are first prepared by grounding into powder. They are then added into the mixture using geometric dilution.

Water-soluble ingredients should first be dissolved in water before being added to the base. After compounding, the mixture should be smooth.

Creams

These are semisolid drug formulations made from water and oil. They are, however, thicker than lotions and can be dispensed from a tube or a jar. They are compounded just as ointments.

Pastes

These are semisolid drug topical formulations. They do not melt at body temperature. They are similar to ointments and creams but have higher quantities of solid particles. They are compounded just as ointments.

Gels

These are semisolid drug formulations made from organic or inorganic molecules. They are compounded like ointments.

Suppositories

These are solid drug formulations made for insertion into orifices. They are locally applied drugs. The bases of these drugs can be made from cocoa butter, which melts at body temperature and is commonly used to make rectal suppositories. Another form of base is Carbowax, also known as polyethylene glycol, which is water-soluble and used for rectal or vaginal suppositories. Glycerinated gelatin is a water-soluble base that is used for vaginal and rectal suppositories. Before compounding a suppository, you must think of the appropriate mold to put it in. Suppository molds come in plastic, rubber, stainless steel or brass.

Capsules

This is a solid drug formulation in which the drug is encased in a soft gelatin gel. The size of capsules ranges from 5 to 000. The largest size an adult can swallow is 0. Capsules are filled through punching. In this method, the drug powder is compressed into the capsule with a spatula. For large-scale productions, capsule filling machines are used.

Tablets

This is a solid drug formulation made by compressing or molding drug powders. These powders are then bound together with water and alcohol. Moistening agents and diluents are used to compound tablets. The mixture is poured into a mold, spread out and then punched. The soft tablets are left to dry out on the peg.

Powders

These are solid drug formulations. They are ideal for administering drugs whose dosages in capsules or tablets will be too large to swallow. They can, however, have an unpleasant taste. Trituration is used to blend the powders. Geometric dilution can also be used. Before mixing powders of different sizes, they should each be reduced either by grinding or crushing.

Mathematics

Formulas

Calculation of drug dosages

The basic formula is:

Amount of drug = $d/h \times v$
Where d is the desired dose to be given, v means the vehicle (the form of the drug dosage and route of administration) and h is the dose on hand (the dose on the label).

Ratio and proportion

$H : V = D : X$
H is the dose on hand. V is the vehicle. D is the desired dose, and X is the amount of drug to be given.

Fractional equation

$H/V = D/X$
H is the dose on hand. V is the vehicle. D is the desired dose, and X is the amount of drug to be given.

Measure oral liquid drugs

$D/H \times V = X$
D is the desired dose to be given. H is the dose on hand. V is the volume of the drug.

Flow rate of IV heparin

$D/H \times Q = R$ (mL/hr)
D is the dose to be given. H is the dose on hand. Q is the amount of heparin available (mL).

Calculation of drop rates

R = V/T × C
R is the flow rate (gtt/min). V is volume to be infused(mL). T is time for the solution to be infused (minutes), and C is drop factor (gtt/mL).

Calculation of pediatric doses

There are different rules used to calculate dosages for pediatric patients. These rules take into consideration the patient's weight, age and body surface area. Even if pediatric doses are calculated in proportion to adult doses, a child is not a miniature adult. Metabolic rates in pediatric and adult patients differ because of the presence of immature/growing organs.

Clark's Rule
Pediatric dose = Weight of the child (pounds)/150 pounds × adult dose.

Fried's Rule – Used for children less than 12 months.
Child's dose = Age of the patient (months)/150 × average adult dose

Young's Rule – Used for children older than 12 months.
Child's dose = (child's age (years)/child's age + 12) × adult dose

To calculate the dose of the drug based on the patient's body surface area:
Pediatric dose = Adult dose × Child's body surface area (m2) /1.7m2

Ratios

It is important to know how to convert ratios to percentages and how to convert ratios from dosages. A ratio is written as 1:1,000, 1:100 and so on. The number on the left side represents values in grams, while the one on the right represents values in milliliters (liquids) and grams (solids). For example, a drug written as 1:10,000 means there is 1 g of drug dissolved in 10,000 mL of solution.

Let's say you get an order in milligrams, and the inventory expresses the drugs in ratio. You should be able to convert the drug in the inventory from ratios to milliliters. For easy recall, always remember that:

1:10 1 g/10 mL
1:100 is 1 g/ 100 mL = 1% solution
1:1,000 is the same as 1 g/ 1000 mL

Percentages
Percentages are used to calculate the number of grams of a drug in 100 mL of a solution or weight per volume (w/v); the amount of grams of a drug in 100 g of a solid or weight per weight (w/w); or the volume of a drug in 100 mL of a solution, which is called volume per volume (v/v).

Alligation
This is used to calculate a mixture of two different solutions that have been mixed to yield another solution with a different percentage.

Conversions

There are three basic measurement systems used in pharmacies. They are:

The household system – This is also known as the Avoirdupois System. It is readily understood by patients because it uses conventional measurements, like tablespoons, gallons, quarts, teaspoons, pints and quarts. This measurement system uses crude estimates and is therefore not used by health-care providers for calculating doses of drugs.

1 tbsp. = 3 tsp
1 oz = 2 tbsp
1 cup = 8 oz

This measurement system lacks uniformity because these measuring containers come in different shapes and sizes.

Conversion factors

Unit of measure	Abbreviation	Conversion
Grains	gr	60 mg – 65 mg
1 teaspoon	1 tsp	5 mL
1 tablespoon	1 tbsp	15 mL
1 pint	1 pt	16 fl. oz
1 quart	1 qt	2 pints
1 gallon	1 gal	4 quarts
1 fluid ounce	fl. oz	30 mL

Metric system – This is the most common system used in pharmacies. It is the legal system for measurement in the United States and most developed nations. Its measurement depends on the decimal system. The three basic units are the gram, liter and meter.

The gram is the basic unit for measuring weight.

1 g = 1 cc/1mL of water
1 g = 15 gr
1 g = 0.034 oz

1 g = 1,000 mg
1 mg = 1000 mcg
1 mg = 0.001 g
1 kg = 1,000 g

The liter is the basic unit for measuring volume.

1 L = 1,000 cc
1 L = 1.056 quarts = 0.26 gallon = 2.1 pints
1 L = 1,000 mL
1 mL = 1 cc = 0.001 L

The meter is used to measure length. It is not used to calculate dosages of drugs but to calculate the height of individuals.

The apothecary system – This system is not common in the United States. It is an old system of measurement. It is also called the US liquid measure system and the wine measure system. This system uses fractions instead of decimals and Roman numerals in place of Arabic numbers. Weight is measured in grain (gr). Dram is another unit for weight.

1 dr = 60 gr
1 oz = 8 dr

The unit of measurement for liquid volume is minim (m). Volume can also be measured in ounces and drams.

International units – This system measures drugs in units (U or IU). Examples of drugs measured with this system include heparin, penicillin G and insulin. It is not necessary to convert the units to milligrams because the amount of drugs in milligrams is not standardized.

Milliequivalents – A milliequivalent is a measure of the amount of positively charged ions present in a liter of salt solution. Milliequivalent (mEq) is used to measure salt solutions like potassium chloride.

1 Eq = 1,000 mEq

Conversion of systems of measurement

CPhTs should be able to convert drugs from one system of measurement to the other. They should also be able to dispense drugs to patients in a measurement system that the patient understands. For example, a physician's prescription written as "10 mL tds" should be translated to the patient as "take two teaspoons three times a day." Conversions are commonly done to the metric system. This requires memorization of conversion tables.

Conversions of temperature

The units of measurement for temperature are Celsius and Fahrenheit. Household scales often use Fahrenheit, while scientific scales use Celsius.

To convert Celsius to Fahrenheit:
°C = (°F-32) × (5/9)

To convert Fahrenheit to Celsius:
°F = °C × (9/5) + 32.

Sig codes

These are abbreviations used for prescribing. Examples include:

q – Every
qAM – Every morning
qH – Every hour
q__° – Hourly
qHS – Every bedtime
qD – Daily
qOD – Alternate day
qMO – monthly
qPM – Every evening
qWK – Weekly
C – With
HS – At bedtime
PRN – As needed
PC – After a meal
q__H – Every – hours
BID – Twice a day
TID – Three times a day
QID – Four times a day
QS – Quantity sufficient
UD – As directed
GTT – Drop
AA – Of each
X_D – Times_day
TDS – Three times a day
AC – Before a meal

Roman numerals

The CPhT should be able to use and interpret Roman numerals because they are used for writing dosages and representing values in measurement systems (apothecary units).

Roman numerals are written and read from left to right in descending order. The placement of the numeral is also important. For example, when the numerals are written in descending order from left to right, they are added into a cumulative number (MC means 1,000 + 100 = 1,100). However, if a numeral with a small value is placed next to a numeral of a large value, it is deducted (CM means 1,000 – 100 = 900).

Equipment/Supplies Required for Drug Administration

Equipment for oral drugs

Medicine cups – These are calibrated cups used to administer large quantities of oral liquid drugs. Cups can be 30 mL or 1 oz. Drugs that are less than 5 mL should be given in another measuring container.

Medicine droppers – These are used to administer smaller drops of liquid drugs to infants and smaller children. Droppers measure medication in drops and milliliters.

Calibrated spoons – These are used to give oral drugs to older children who are more cooperative and less fussy. They are calibrated from one-fourth teaspoon (about 1 cc) to two teaspoons (10 cc).

Equipment for parenteral administration

Needles – Needles can be disposable or nondisposable. Sizes of the needle gauge range from 13 to 31 G. The length of the needle varies from three-eighth inches to two inches. The parts of a needle include the bevel, shaft and hub.

Syringes – Syringes can be disposable or nondisposable. Disposable syringes are nontoxic, sterilized, prepackaged and ready for use. Sizes of syringes range from 0.5 to 60 cc. They can be prefilled or hypodermic.

Hypodermic syringes are used for subcutaneous and IV and IM injections. They are available in sizes ranging from 1 to 60 cc. Lager-sized syringes are used to prepare IV drugs for administration. Types of hypodermic syringes include:

Needleless syringes – Needleless syringes use a jet injector and high pressure to deliver injections.

Insulin syringes – Insulin syringes are used to deliver insulin. They are calibrated in units (U or UI). They can be U-40 or U-100 and come in sizes 1 cc, 0.3 cc and 0.5 cc.

Tuberculin syringes – Tuberculin syringes are used to administer small volumes of parenteral drugs, usually less than or equal to 1 mL.

Prefilled syringes are also called cartridges. They are disposable, sterilized and ready for one-time use.

Medication containers

Ampoules – These are small glass containers that have been hermetically sealed. There are scoured weak points on their necks that make it easy to break to extract the drug.

Vials – These are small bottles that have rubber stoppers. To extract the drug, an injection is passed through the stopper. Vials can be a single dose or multidose. It is important to use a sterile single-use syringe to extract drugs from a multidose vial. This act reduces the risk of contaminating the vial and infecting patients. Vials can contain as much as 100 mL of the drug.

How to give oral drugs

Before administering an oral drug, confirm if it should be taken on an empty or full stomach.

Capsules and pills should be taken with water. Some fluids can aid or block the absorption of certain drugs. For example, orange juice improves the absorption of iron; milk, on the other hand, prevents the absorption of antibiotics like fluoroquinolones. Taking sildenafil with grapefruit juice can cause serious side effects, like shock. Capsules and tablets should not be chewed, broken or crushed.

Pay attention to patients who complain of difficulty swallowing. Another form of oral administration should be considered (liquids).

Liquid medications are ideal for children because they are easy to swallow, especially if the drug is sweetened and enhanced with flavors.

Before administering a liquid drug, be sure to shake well. Calibrated containers—like spoons, droppers and cups—should be used.

Sublingual and buccal drugs should not be chewed or crushed. Chewable tablets, on the other hand, should not be swallowed.

Lozenges should be sucked on. They should not be swallowed or chewed.

Lot Numbers

This is an identification number printed on medications to help manufacturers identify drug batches. Lot numbers make it possible for the calculation of expiration dates, drug recalls and quality control. Lot numbers are printed on drug labels, next to expiration dates and barcodes.

Lot tracking

This is a quality control method in which drug manufacturers track drugs with their lot numbers. Lot tracking is useful for maintaining supply chain integrity and managing inventory. By storing production information on lot numbers, manufacturers can track even the raw materials used in making drugs.

Lot tracking is also used to determine the batches of drugs that are up for sale, locate expired batches and find batches that need to be recalled. Lot tracking also makes root-cause analysis easier because it provides information on the raw materials and the manufacturing process.

Lot tracking improves the integrity of the supply chain because it makes it easy to trace the pedigree of drug batches. This simply means that lot tracking makes it easier to track down the ingredients and dosages of different drug batches from production to processing and distribution.

Expiration dates and testing

The FDA requires all OTC drugs, insulin products and prescription drugs to have expiration dates. Expiration dates are determined by stability testing. The test is done to assess the ideal storage requirements and expiration dates.

Requirements for this test include:

1. Provision of test intervals and sample size
2. Use of reliable and sensitive testing methods
3. Provision of closure systems similar to the ones used for marketing
4. Testing of drugs before and after they are reconstituted
5. Expiration dates do not apply to damaged or defective drugs because expiration dates depend on storage conditions.
6. Drugs with earlier expiration dates should be stocked in front of drugs with later expiration dates. This is known as the First Expired, First Out strategy.

National Drug Code (NDC) numbers

The FDA assigns these numbers for quality control and improvement. It is a set of 10 to 11 numbers given to drug manufacturers of prescription medicines, insulin products and OTC drugs to monitor how these drugs are manufactured, salvaged, distributed and packaged. Companies expected to obey this law are foreign and domestic drug manufacturers, relabelers, repackers and salvagers, private label distributors and companies involved in salvaging, repackaging, relabeling and manufacturing biologic agents.

Procedures for Identifying and Returning Dispensable, Non-dispensable and Expired Medications and Supplies

Expired drugs

The CPhT should check the stock once a month for expired or soon-to-expire drugs (in the next two or three months). These drugs should be promptly removed from the stock. Wholesalers can accept expired drugs on credit only if they are returned within a certain period, most times two or three months before they are expired. To do so, the CPhT will first create a list of the names of the drugs to be returned, including their dosages, strengths, quantities and formations. This list is forwarded to the wholesaler for review.

After approval by the wholesaler, the drugs are packaged and shipped. It is important that the CPhT inspect the stock and consult the wholesalers before the drugs expire and the pharmacy runs at a loss. In cases where the drugs are unacceptable by the wholesaler, they can be sent to a reverse distributor on credit.

Reverse distributors collect and process damaged, recalled and expired drugs from pharmacies and send them back to the drug manufacturers. In exchange for their services, they collect a percentage out of the refund sent to the pharmacy. Partially used drugs and reconstituted and compounded drugs are usually not accepted by drug manufacturers.

Overstock returns

Drugs that have been ordered in excess quantities can be returned to the wholesaler. For this to happen, the CPhT should inspect the stock for products that are not selling as they should. The wholesaler should be contacted for approval for a return, and the names of the drugs should be sent. As soon as the approval is granted, the drugs should be packaged and shipped to the wholesaler.

Damaged drugs

When the CPhT receives drugs into the stock, they should be inspected. Damaged drugs should be returned for replacement, provided they have not been used. The

CPhT contacts the wholesaler and sends a list of the defective drugs for approval. If approval is granted, the wholesaler sends a return form or an approval code.

Test 1: Questions

1. Which of the following is false about the chemical name of a drug?
   A. It is also called the scientific name.
   B. It is used in conventional language.
   C. The most important naming system is the IUPAC name.
   D. Drugs are named according to the structure of the drug molecules.

2. Which of the following is a generic name?
   A. Penicillin
   B. Advil
   C. N-acetyl-p-aminophenol
   D. Zoloft

3. Which of the following is another name for the brand name of a drug?
   A. Proprietary name
   B. Scientific name
   C. Trademark name
   D. Copyright name

4. According to the ATC system, level 1 classifies drugs according to __________.
   A. Therapeutic action
   B. Organ systems
   C. Mechanism of action
   D. Chemical properties

5. Which of the following levels of the ATC system classifies drugs according to chemical components?
   A. Level 2
   B. Level 3
   C. Level 4
   D. Level 5

6. Drugs with no risk of teratogenicity are grouped into which of the following categories?

A. Category X
B. Category N
C. Category A
D. Category D

7. Which of the following pregnancy categories describes drugs that have not yet been categorized by the FDA?

A. Category X
B. Category N
C. Category A
D. Category D

8. Which of the following best describes drugs in pregnancy Category X?

A. Drugs that have well-controlled human trials and animal trials that have shown fetal risks, adverse reactions and fetal abnormalities
B. Drugs with demonstrated risk to the human fetus but that can be used if the benefits outweigh the risks to the fetus
C. Drugs with adverse effects demonstrated in animal trials but with insufficient data on well-controlled trials in pregnant women
D. Drugs with no fetal risk demonstrated during animal trials, with insufficient well-controlled human trials. It also includes drugs that have demonstrated adverse fetal risks in animal trials but that have not demonstrated risks to the fetus in well-controlled human trials.

9. Which of the following is false about Schedule I drugs?

A. They have a high potential for abuse and addiction.
B. They are safe for medical use only under strict medical supervision.
C. Heroin is an example.
D. Psilocybin is an example.

10. Which of the following is a Schedule II drug?
   A. Mescaline
   B. Cathinone
   C. Phencyclidine
   D. Ketamine

11. Concerning LASA medications, what is the most appropriate description?
   A. Medications that have similarities in shape only
   B. Medications that have similarities in name only
   C. Medications that appear similar in chemical properties
   D. Medications that are similar in physical structure, packaging and drug names with similar spellings or pronunciation

12. Which of the following is not a risk factor associated with LASA medications?
   A. Illegible writing
   B. Incomplete knowledge of drug names
   C. Medications with different clinical uses
   D. Similar packaging and label

13. Which of the following is a strategy used to reduce error during procurement of LASA medications?
   A. Tall man lettering
   B. Encouraging the availability of multiple medicine strengths
   C. Reducing the availability of multiple medicine strengths
   D. Additional warning labels

14. The act of writing part of the name of a medication in upper case to help differentiate LASA medications is called ___________________.
   A. Slow man lettering
   B. Upper case lettering
   C. Legible writing
   D. Tall man lettering

15. Which of the following is not an example of drug pairs with tall man lettering?

A. metFORMIN and metoPROLOL
B. nitroGLYCERINe and nitroPRUSSIDe
C. LOsartan and LOvastatin
D. ACETAminophen and ACETALdehyde

16. Which of the following is false about the metric system of measurement?

A. It is commonly used at home.
B. It is the legal system of measurement in the United States.
C. It uses the decimal system.
D. It includes the gram, meter and liter.

17. Which of the following measurement systems is also known as the Avoirdupois System?

A. The metric system
B. The international unit system
C. The household system
D. The apothecary system

18. Which of the following statements is false concerning triangle checks in LASA medications?

A. You should check the actual medicines against the medication label.
B. You should check the actual medications against the prescription.
C. You should identify medication only by physical appearance.
D. It is done during administration and dispensation of drugs.

19. Concerning patient education on medications, which of the following is false?

A. The patient should be informed of changes in the appearance of medication.
B. Patients and caregivers should inform the health-care provider if the medication appears different from what is usually administered.
C. Patients and caregivers should be encouraged to learn the names of their medication.
D. Patients should be encouraged to perform a triangle check before taking their medication.

20. Concerning the monitoring of LASA medication, which of the following is incorrect?

A. All facilities should identify medications that look or sound alike in their organization.
B. Periodic reviews and updates of the LASA list should be performed.
C. Feedback mechanisms to provide information on LASA medication should be implemented.
D. Staff should be informed of medications listed as LASA only once a year.

21. Which of the following best describes a Class A prescription balance?

A. A device used to measure large quantities of material and drugs above 5 kg
B. A balance that is usually composed of a single pan
C. A measuring device used to weigh quantities that are not more than 120 g
D. A balance used for mixing certain compounds

22. Concerning conical graduates, which of the following is true?
   A. They are used in the measurement of liquids that have wide bases and wide tops and taper from the top to bottom.
   B. They are useful when measuring liquids that have narrow diameters at the top and base.
   C. They are usually in the form of plates made up of hard, flat and nonabsorbent surfaces.
   D. They are used in the measurement of solid drugs.

23. Which of the following may be referred to as compounding?
1 – Preparation of radioactive isotopes
2 – Preparation of suppositories, oral liquids and topical medications
3 – Conversion from one dosage form to another
   A. 2 only
   B. 2 and 3
   C. 3 only
   D. 1, 2 and 3

24. Which of the following materials is incorrectly paired with its use?
   A. Heat guns – Used to shrink bands onto vials
   B. Decappers – Used to remove seals on containers
   C. Beakers – Used to hold liquids
   D. Hot plates – Used for drying tablets during compounding

25. Which of the following is true about formulating suspensions?
   A. It is easy to maintain the physical stability of suspensions after compounding.
   B. It does not require the process of trituration.
   C. Suspensions are difficult to compound.
   D. A suspension is a heterogeneous mixture.

26. Which of the following is correct about the compounding of suspensions?
   A. Suspensions are not filtered.
   B. Suspensions are combined with a low-speed mixer.
   C. A light-sensitive bottle is used to store suspensions.
   D. Levigating agents are added quickly.

27. Which of the following is correct regarding solutions?
   A. They require shaking before use.
   B. Sterile solutions include oral and otic solutions.
   C. The solubility characteristic of each active ingredient must be known.
   D. All active ingredients in a solution must be dissolved in the same solvent.

28. Which of the following is not a property of elixirs?
   A. They need to be stirred continuously during preparation.
   B. Alcohol required for an elixir is usually minimal.
   C. They are compounded by combining different kinds of alcohol with sugar.
   D. They are compounded by combining alcohol-soluble and water-soluble ingredients.

29. Which of the following statements concerning an emulsion is true?
   A. An emulsion is a type of solution.
   B. Oil-in-water emulsions are not greasy.
   C. Water-in-oil emulsions are not greasy.
   D. Water-in-oil emulsions are usually for oral use.

30. Which of the following statements is false regarding the compounding of emulsions?
   A. There are four methods for compounding emulsions.
   B. The dry gum method of compounding is also known as the continental method.
   C. The continental method is the preferred method of compounding emulsions.
   D. In the English method, gum acacia is first combined with an oil.

31. Which of the following is true concerning the labeling of controlled substances?

A. Drug manufacturers are required by federal law to use a particular symbol to indicate that it is a controlled substance.
B. A container of a patient's medication should carry a message prohibiting the transfer of medication.
C. A Schedule III controlled substance is denoted as CIII.
D. All of the above.

32. Which of the following is correct regarding the FDA drug risk management process?

A. The FDA considers a drug to be safe if the benefits of using it outweigh the risk.
B. The FDA considers a drug to be safe if it has no adverse effects.
C. The FDA considers a drug to be safe if it is used by a large population.
D. The FDA considers a drug to be safe if it is used for terminally ill patients.

33. At what stage of the drug risk management process are determinations made to assess if the benefits of taking a drug outweigh the risk?

A. Assessment
B. Making adjustments
C. Evaluating effectiveness
D. Minimizing

34. Which of the following is not part of the process of drug risk management?

A. Assessment
B. Minimizing
C. Optimization
D. Evaluating effectiveness

35. The risk evaluation and management strategy (REM) is used to achieve all except ____________.

A. Eliminating the risk associated with taking certain drugs
B. Closely monitoring patients who take REM drugs
C. Educating health-care providers and pharmacists
D. Providing specific requirements on the use of certain drugs

36. A drug used in the treatment of patients requires risk evaluation and management monitoring to monitor its effects on the patient population. Which of the following drugs requires REM monitoring?

A. Acetaminophen
B. Lemtrada
C. Vasoprin
D. Vasopressin

37. Which of the following is not a factor considered by the FDA before it requires REM for a drug?

A. How new the drug is
B. How often adverse effects have occurred within a population
C. The size of the population to use the drug
D. The strength of drug dosage

38. Which of the following ingredients is present in OTC cold medications but is also used in the illegal manufacturing of street drugs?

A. Methamphetamine
B. Pseudoephedrine
C. Epinephrine
D. Latruda

39. Which of the following drugs is used in the treatment of type 1 diabetes mellitus?

A. Metformin
B. Glyburide
C. Glipizide
D. Humulin

40. You are to give an IV drug to a child. If the adult dose is 20 mg/kg and the child weighs 30 kg, what is the dose to be given to this child?

A. 150 mg
B. 600 mg
C. 300 mg
D. 400 mg

41. You are to give an IM drug to a child. If the adult dose is 15 mg/kg and the child weighs 60 lbs, what is the dose to be given to this child?

A. 365 mg
B. 450 mg
C. 409 mg
D. 200 mg

42. You are to give a drug to a five-year-old child who weighs 50 lbs. If the adult dose of the drug is 200 mg, calculate the dose to be given to the child using Young's Rule.

A. 90 mg
B. 120 mg
C. 67 mg
D. 74 mg

43. What dose will be given to the above-mentioned child using Clark's Rule?

A. 90 mg
B. 120 mg
C. 67 mg
D. 74 mg

44. You are to give a drug at the rate of 40 mg/m2 to a child who weighs 66 pounds and is 42 inches tall. What dose of the drug will be given?

A. 38 mg
B. 45 mg
C. 101 mg
D. 201 mg

45. You are to give a drug at the rate of 60 mg/m2 to a child who weighs 50 kg and is 110 cm tall. What dose of the drug will be given?

A. 100 mg
B. 74 mg
C. 200 mg
D. 240 mg

46. You are to give an IV drug to a child. If the adult dose is 10 mg/kg and the child weighs 15 kg, what is the dose to be given to this child?

A. 150 mg
B. 225 mg
C. 15 mg
D. 1.5 mg

47. You are to give a drug to a 10-year-old child who weighs 100 lbs. If the adult dose of the drug is 500 mg, calculate the dose to be given to the child using Young's Rule.

A. 227 mg
B. 500 mg
C. 333 mg
D. 450 mg

48. You are to give a drug to a 10-year-old child who weighs 100 lbs. If the adult dose of the drug is 500 mg, calculate the dose to be given to the child using Clark's Rule.

A. 227 mg
B. 500 mg
C. 333 mg
D. 450 mg

49. Which of the following is a Schedule IV drug?

A. Tramadol
B. Codeine
C. Hydromorphone
D. Psilocybin

50. Which of the following is false about therapeutic equivalence between two drugs?

A. The two drugs must contain the same active ingredients.
B. They must be FDA approved.
C. They must have the same packaging.
D. They must have the same pharmacokinetics.

51. Which of the following best describes pharmaceutical equivalence?

A. Drugs with the same bioavailability
B. Drugs with the same active ingredient but expressed in different esters
C. Drugs with the same pharmacokinetics and pharmacodynamics
D. Drugs with a different mechanism of action but treat the same disease condition

52. Which of the following describes a drug's ability to act on a receptor site?

A. Affinity
B. Selectivity
C. Residence time
D. Intrinsic efficacy

53. Which of the following describes the likelihood of a drug occupying a receptor?

A. Affinity
B. Selectivity
C. Residence time
D. Intrinsic efficacy

54. Which of the following describes a drug that acts as an antagonist only in the presence of other agonists?

A. Reverse agonist
B. Partial agonist
C. Competitive antagonist
D. Noncompetitive antagonist

55. Which of the following is false about passive diffusion across membranes?
   A. Substances move from an area of high concentration to an area of low concentration.
   B. Water-soluble molecules diffuse quickly.
   C. Small molecules diffuse quickly.
   D. Un-ionized molecules diffuse quickly.

56. Which of the following statements is false about facilitated diffusion?
   A. It occurs toward a concentration gradient.
   B. Lipids are transported by this means.
   C. It does not require energy.
   D. Diffusion is done via carrier molecules.

57. What form of cellular transport requires energy to transport molecules against a concentration gradient?
   A. Pinocytosis
   B. Active transport
   C. Facilitated diffusion
   D. Passive diffusion

58. Concerning the oral administration of drugs, which of the following statements is correct?
   A. The stomach has a large surface area and a long transit time.
   B. Drugs are mostly absorbed in the large intestine.
   C. Food delays gastric emptying.
   D. The stomach has a thin mucosa.

59. Which of the following options is the most appropriate reason for the classification of a drug as a high-alert medication?
   A. The drug looks like other drugs.
   B. It is very expensive.
   C. It requires high doses to achieve a therapeutic effect.
   D. It has a narrow therapeutic index.

60. Which of the following classes of drugs is not a high-alert medication?

A. Insulin
B. Anticoagulants
C. Nonsteroidal anti-inflammatory drugs (NSAIDs)
D. Narcotics

61. Concerning high-alert medications, which of the following is not true?

A. High-alert medications have a narrow therapeutic margin.
B. Little dosage or blood concentration changes can cause serious dose or blood-concentration critical events.
C. Adverse effects can be life-threatening and require hospitalization.
D. An example is acetaminophen.

62. Which of the following is not useful in preventing errors of insulin administration?

A. Separate insulin vials from heparin vials.
B. Avoid abbreviations.
C. Implement a check-and-balance system.
D. Store insulin in the fridge.

63. Hypertonic sodium chloride is a high-alert drug because it increases the risk of ______________.

A. Cerebral edema
B. Pulmonary edema
C. Phlebitis
D. Liver failure

64. What term is used to describe a patient's ability to be free from injuries caused by medical care?

A. Patient safety
B. Patient freedom
C. Medication error
D. Prescription error

65. Which of the following strategies is not useful in reducing the risk of errors when administering heparin?

A. Use single-dose vials.
B. Use commercially available premixes.
C. Use standardized concentrations.
D. Store heparin vials away from insulin vials.

66. Which of the following is not a withdrawal symptom of benzodiazepine abuse?

A. Hyperpyrexia
B. Tachycardia
C. Seizures
D. Diarrhea

67. Which of the following vaccine reactions is caused by the properties of a vaccine?

A. Vaccine quality defect–related reaction
B. Vaccine product–related reaction
C. Coincidental event
D. Immunization error–related reactions

68. All these increase the risk of human error during prescription except?

A. Fatigue
B. Poor lighting
C. Noise
D. Barcode

69. Concerning the formulation of pastes, which of the following is true?

A. All pastes contain a medication.
B. Pastes contain a higher amount of solids than creams.
C. Pastes soften at body temperature.
D. Pastes are compounded through a more complex technique than ointments.

70. Which of the following is false about the production of gels?
  A. They are compounded using inorganic or organic particles.
  B. Actions result in local effects.
  C. They are generally applied locally.
  D. They do not bring about systemic effects.

71. Which of the following statements is false about creams?
  A. Usually, creams are for topical use.
  B. They are compounded in the same manner as ointments.
  C. They do not contain medication.
  D. They are a combination of water and oil.

72. Concerning the formulation of ointments, which of the following is false?
  A. Ointments are water-based products.
  B. Insoluble powders may be used during their compounding.
  C. The final product should be smooth and free of abrasive particles.
  D. Drugs in the form of crystals or powders may be compounded into ointments.

73. Which of the following materials is least useful for compounding ointments?
  A. A glass slab
  B. A spatula
  C. A tablet mold
  D. A mortar

74. Suppositories can be produced using all except ___________ as bases.
  A. Cocoa butter
  B. Almond butter
  C. Glycerinated gelatin
  D. Polyethylene glycol

75. All except which of these factors affect the rate of distribution of a drug?
   A. Permeability of the membranes
   B. Tissue binding
   C. Receptor affinity
   D. Regional pH

76. Concerning the volume of distribution of a drug, which of the following is false?
   A. The apparent volume of distribution is theoretical.
   B. Acidic drugs have large volumes of distribution.
   C. Basic drugs have large volumes of distribution.
   D. Acidic drugs are readily bound to proteins.

77. Concerning the binding of drugs, which of the following statements is false?
   A. Acidic drugs readily bind to albumin.
   B. Basic drugs readily bind to adipose tissue.
   C. Unbound drugs are transported by passive diffusion.
   D. The therapeutic effect of a drug is carried out by its unbound molecules.

78. Drugs do not readily enter the brain because of the blood-brain barrier. Which of the following is not a component of the blood-brain barrier?
   A. Endothelial cells
   B. Astrocytic sheath
   C. Choroid plexus
   D. Basement membrane

79. Which of the following does not affect a drug's rate of metabolism?
   A. Genetics
   B. Liver diseases
   C. Drug interactions
   D. The drug's pH

80. In which order of kinetics is the rate of metabolism proportional to the amount of unmetabolized drugs left?

A. First order
B. Second order
C. Zero order
D. Third order

81. Which of the following reactions occurs in phase I metabolism?

A. Hydrolysis
B. Oxidation
C. Glucuronidation
D. Conjugation

82. Which of the following reactions occurs in phase II metabolism?

A. Hydrolysis
B. Oxidation
C. Glucuronidation
D. Conjugation

83. Which of the following is the primary route of drug excretion?

A. Urine
B. Saliva
C. Feces
D. Sweat

84. Concerning the renal excretion of drugs, which of the following statements is false?

A. Metabolites are conjugated into salts to make them water-soluble.
B. Acidifying the urine increases the rate of excretion of weak acids.
C. Inhibitors can block the excretion of metabolites by acting on the proximal convoluted tubule.
D. Renal excretion decreases with age.

85. You are counseling Mrs. Philips, a 65-year-old female on aspirin for myocardial infarction, to avoid taking ibuprofen for her knee pain to prevent the risk of myocardial infarction. Which of the following best describes the mechanism of this drug-drug interaction?

A. Aspirin prevents the metabolism of ibuprofen.
B. Ibuprofen blocks prostaglandin synthesis.
C. Aspirin increases the excretion of ibuprofen.
D. Ibuprofen competes with aspirin for the COX-1 receptor.

86. Mr. Phelps, a 56-year-old male on citalopram for a depressive disorder, presents to the pharmacy for ibuprofen, an OTC. You know that a drug-drug interaction between an SSRI and an NSAID increases the risk of gastrointestinal bleeding. Which of the following best describes the mechanism of citalopram in causing the bleeding?

A. It binds to COX-1 and blocks platelet aggregation.
B. It competes with ibuprofen for the COX-1 receptor.
C. It prevents the reuptake of serotonin in dopaminergic neurons.
D. It blocks the transport of serotonin into platelets.

87. All except which of the following drug-drug interactions increases the risk of gastrointestinal bleeding?

A. SSRI and NSAID
B. SSRI and warfarin
C. NSAID and ACEI
D. Warfarin and erythromycin

88. A drug interaction with sertraline and sumatriptan will increase the risk of

______________.

A. Coagulopathies
B. Serotonin syndrome
C. Hypertension
D. Hyperkalemia

89. Which of the following drug-drug interactions will increase the risk of Torsade de Pointes?

A. Fluoroquinolone and erythromycin
B. Citalopram and diclofenac
C. Warfarin and Amiodarone
D. Spironolactone and eplerenone

90. Antacids containing calcium carbonate block the absorption of all except which of the following drugs in the gut?

A. Tetracycline
B. Iron
C. Levothyroxine
D. Citalopram

Test 1: Answers and Explanations

1. (B) It is used in conventional language.
This statement is false. The chemical name is also known as the scientific name. In this system of naming, drugs are named according to how the drug's molecules are structured. The most important chemical naming system for drugs is the International Union of Pure and Applied Chemistry (IUPAC) naming system. Chemical names are long and often difficult to remember. They are not used in conventional language.

2. (A) Penicillin.
Generic names are used for drug groups with similar actions. They are useful in identifying the class of a drug and its active ingredient. Generic names are also called nonproprietary names. Examples include penicillin, atorvastatin, sertraline, etc. Option B is a brand name. Option C is a chemical name, and Option D is a brand name.

3. (C) Trademark name.
Brand names are also called trademark names. Trademark names are names given by pharmaceutical companies to drugs that have been tried, tested and approved by regulatory bodies. A lot of drugs have multiple trademark names that differ from country to country.

4. (B) Organ systems.
Level 1 (organ system) – Drugs are classified according to the system of the body receiving the therapeutic effects. There are 14 letters.

Level 2 (therapeutic action) – This is made up of two digits and describes the drug's therapeutic action.

Level 3 (mechanism of action) – Drugs are grouped according to their mechanism of action. This classification is made up of a letter.

Level 4 (chemical properties) – Drugs are grouped according to their pharmacological or chemical property. This classification is made up of a letter.

Level 5 (chemical components) – Drugs are grouped according to their chemical components or substances. This classification is made up of two digits.

5. (D) Level 5.
Level 5 (chemical components) – Drugs are grouped according to their chemical components or substances. This classification is made up of two digits.

6. (C) Category A.
Category A includes drugs with no risks demonstrated during controlled human trials. Trials did not show risks to fetuses during the first trimester or later trimesters of pregnancy.

7. (B) Category N.
Category N includes drugs that have not yet been classified by the FDA into a pregnancy category.

8. (A) Drugs that have well-controlled human trials and animal trials that have shown fetal risks, adverse reactions and fetal abnormalities.
Category X drugs are contraindicated in pregnancy. Well-controlled human trials and animal trials have shown fetal risks, adverse reactions and fetal abnormalities. The drugs have risks that outweigh their benefits.

9. (B) They are safe for medical use only under strict medical supervision.
This statement is false because Schedule I drugs are not used for any medical conditions. They are unsafe for use even under the strictest medical supervision.

10. (C) Phencyclidine.

Phencyclidine is a Schedule II drug. Other examples of Schedule II drugs are amphetamines, cocaine, barbiturates, pure codeine, fentanyl, hydrocodone, pure diphenoxylate, hydromorphone, morphine, cannabinoids, oxycodone, oxymorphone, methylphenidate, nabilone and pethidine. Options A and B are Schedule I drugs, while Option D is a Schedule III drug.

11. (D) Medications that are similar in physical structure, packaging and drug names with similar spellings or pronunciations.
Look-alike soundalike drugs have similar physical structure, packaging, spellings and pronunciations. These drugs may cause medication errors, and care must be taken to prevent such errors.

12. (C) Medications with different clinical uses.
This is not a risk factor associated with LASA medications. These medications are prone to medication errors due to certain factors. These include illegible writing on prescription orders, which makes it difficult to decipher drug names; incomplete knowledge of the drug names; medications with the same clinical use or that are used in the treatment of some ailments; similar packaging and label; newly available drug products; and drugs with similar strengths, dosage forms, frequency and route of administration.

13. (C) Reducing the availability of multiple medicine strengths.
To avoid medication errors during procurement of LASA drugs, the availability of multiple medicine strengths should be reduced, and the purchase of drugs with similar packaging should be avoided. New products or packaging should also be compared with existing packaging.

14. (D) Tall man lettering.
Tall man lettering is the practice of writing part of the name of a medication in upper case to help differentiate LASA medications and reduce medication errors.

15. (D) ACETAminophen and ACETALdehyde.

This is not an example of a drug pair with tall man lettering. Tall man lettering is used to prevent medication errors that can occur in LASA medications. All the other options are examples of drug pairs with tall man lettering.

16. (A) It is commonly used at home.
This statement is false. The metric system is the most common system used in pharmacies. It is the legal system for measurement in the United States and most developed nations. The apothecary system is commonly used at home.

17. (C) The household system.
The household system is also known as the Avoirdupois System. It is readily understood by patients because it uses conventional measurements like tablespoons, gallons, teaspoons, pints and quarts. This measurement system uses crude estimates and is therefore not used by health-care providers for calculating doses of drugs.

18. (C) You should identify medication only by physical appearance.
This is false. A triangle check involves checking actual medications against the medication label and prescription. It can be performed in the administration and dispensing stages of drug management. Drugs are not only identified by appearance but by labels and drug information too.

19. (D) Patients should be encouraged to perform a triangle check before taking their medication.
This is false. A triangle check is the job of the pharmacist and CPhT. Patient education on medications includes informing patients of changes in the appearance of medication, instructing patients and caregivers to alert health-care personnel if medication appears different and encouraging patients to know the names of their medication.

20. (D) Staff should be informed of medications listed as LASA only once a year.
This statement is false because updates are done periodically, not only on a yearly basis.

21. (C) A measuring device used to weigh quantities that are not more than 120 g.
A Class A prescription balance is used for the measurement of small amounts of drugs and has a maximum capacity of 120 g. It is a two-pan device with a sensitivity requirement of 6 mg.

22. (A) They are used in the measurement of liquids that have wide bases and wide tops and taper from the top to bottom.
Conical graduates are calibrated, cone-shaped tubes usually made of nonabsorbent material. They are useful when measuring liquid substances that have wide bases and wide tops and taper from the top to the bottom.

23. (D) 1, 2 and 3.
Compounding may be described differently by different pharmacists. It may also refer to the conversion from one dose or dosage form into another, the preparation of specific doses from bulk chemicals and the preparation of drugs in syringes, cassettes and other devices for home setting administration.

24. (D) Hot plates – Used for drying tablets during compounding.
This material is incorrectly paired with its use. Hot plates resemble weighing scales and are used for quick heating of substances. Some hot plates are designed with a technique for stirring a substance during heating. Their designs vary for use with either low heat or high heat.

25. (D) A suspension is a heterogeneous mixture.
A suspension is a heterogeneous mixture of solid drug particles and a liquid medium. Suspensions are usually easy to compound. However, maintaining their physical stability after compounding may be a challenge. During their production, the insoluble solids are reduced to fine powder by friction in a process known as trituration, after which a small portion of the liquid is added.

26. (A) Suspensions are not filtered.
This is correct. Suspensions are not filtered after compounding. Levigating agents are liquids used to grind triturated powders to a smooth paste. They

are usually added slowly and mixed into the suspension using a high-speed mixer, after which the suspension is transferred to a light-resistant bottle for dispensing.

27. (C) The solubility characteristic of each active ingredient must be known.
This is correct. The solubility characteristic of each active ingredient required to compound a solution must be known so that ingredients can be dissolved in the appropriate solvents. A solution is a homogenous mixture of a solute and a solvent, so it does not require shaking before use. Sterile solutions include ophthalmic and parenteral solutions. Otic solutions are nonsterile.

28. (D) They are compounded by combining alcohol-soluble and water-soluble ingredients.
This is not a property of elixirs. Elixirs are sweetened liquids made up of water and alcohol. Water-soluble ingredients are first dissolved in water, while alcohol-soluble ingredients are dissolved in alcohol, and the two solvents are then combined. Elixirs require continuous stirring during preparation, and the alcohol concentration should remain as strong as possible.

29. (B) Oil-in-water emulsions are not greasy.
This is true. An emulsion is a type of suspension consisting of two varying liquids and an emulsifier, which holds them together. Water-in-oil emulsions are greasy and used topically, while oil-in-water emulsions are not greasy and usually are for oral use.

30. (A) There are four methods for compounding emulsions.
This is false. There are two methods for producing emulsions, the wet gum (English) method and the dry gum (continental) method. This latter method is preferred for compounding emulsions and involves combining gum acacia and a selected oil first, then adding the desired amount of water and triturating the mixture until its sound and color change.

31. (D) All of the above.
This is true. The labeling of controlled substances is regulated by federal law. It requires that manufacturers use a particular symbol to indicate that the

substance is controlled, and the container of the patient's medication must carry a message to prohibit the transfer of medication. A Schedule III controlled substance is denoted as CIII.

32. (A) The FDA considers a drug to be safe if the benefits of using it outweigh the risks. This is correct. Using the risk management process, the FDA considers a drug to be safe when the benefits of using a drug outweigh its risks.

33. (A) Assessment.
In the assessment stage of drug risk management, a drug is evaluated to see if the benefits of the drug outweigh the risks.

34. (C) Optimization.
Optimization is not part of the drug risk management process. The process is made up of four parts—assessment, making adjustments, evaluating the effectiveness and minimizing.

35. (A) Eliminating the risk associated with taking certain drugs.
REM reduces but does not eliminate the risk of taking certain drugs. It closely monitors patients on REM drugs, provides education to health-care providers and pharmacists and provides specific requirements on the use of certain drugs.

36. (B) Lemtrada.
Lemtrada is a drug used in the treatment of multiple sclerosis. It requires REM. It is given as an IV injection and can cause various adverse effects. Its adverse effects include cerebrovascular accidents, pneumonitis, autoimmune dysfunction and cancer.

37. (D) The strength of drug dosage.
The factors considered by the FDA before requiring REM monitoring include how new a drug is, the incidence of adverse effects that have occurred within a population, the size of the population to use the drug and the duration for

which the patient is to use the drug. The factors do not include the strength of drug dosage.

38. (B) Pseudoephedrine.
Pseudoephedrine is an ingredient present in over-the-counter cold medications. It is used to produce a dangerous and illegal street drug called methamphetamine, a potent drug of abuse that causes physical and psychological dependence.

39. (D) Humulin.
Diabetes mellitus causes elevated blood glucose levels due to relative insulin deficiency, resistance or both. Type 1 insulin is also known as insulin-dependent diabetes mellitus and can be managed using humulin, a form of intermediate-acting human insulin that is available as a subcutaneous injection.

40. (B) 600 mg.
30 kg × 20 mg/kg = 600 mg

41. (C) 409 mg.
First, convert pounds to kg.
60 lbs / 2.2 = 27.3 kg
27.3 kg × 15 mg/kg = 409 mg

42. (D) 74 mg.
According to Young's Rule:
Child's dose = (child's age (years)/child's age + 12) × adult dose
Child's dose = (7/7 + 12) × 200 mg
Child's dose = 73.68 mg = 74 mg

43. (C) 67 mg.
According to Clark's Rule:
Child's dose = weight of child (lbs)/150) × adult dose
Child's dose = (50 lbs/150) × 200 mg
Child's dose = 66.67 mg = 67 mg

44. (A) 38 mg.
First, calculate the BSA of the patient.
$\text{BSA} = \sqrt{(\text{pounds} \times \text{inches})} / \sqrt{3{,}131}$
$\text{BSA} = \sqrt{(2{,}772)} / \sqrt{3{,}131}$
$\text{BSA} = 52.65/55.96$
$\text{BSA} = 0.94 \text{ m2}$
$0.94 \times 40 \text{ mg/m2} = 37.63 \text{ mg} = 38 \text{ mg}$

45. (B) 74 mg.
First, calculate the BSA of the patient.
$\text{BSA} = \sqrt{(\text{kg} \times \text{cm})} / \sqrt{3{,}600}$
$\text{BSA} = \sqrt{5{,}500} / \sqrt{3{,}600}$
$\text{BSA} = 74.16/60$
$\text{BSA} = 1.236$
$1.236 \times 60 \text{ mg/m2} = 74.16 \text{ mg} = 74 \text{ mg}$

46. (A) 150 mg.
$15 \text{ kg} \times 10 \text{ mg/kg} = 150 \text{ mg}$

47. (A) 227 mg.
According to Young's Rule:
Child's dose = (child's age (years)/child's age + 12) × adult dose
Child's dose = (10/10 + 12) × 500 mg
Child's dose = 0.45 × 500 mg
Child's dose = 227 mg

48. (C) 333 mg.
According to Clark's Rule:
Child's dose = weight of child (lbs)/150) × adult dose
Child's dose = (100 lbs/150) × 500 mg
Child's dose = (0.67) × 500 mg
Child's dose = 333 mg

49. (A) Tramadol.

Tramadol is a Schedule IV drug. Option B is a Schedule V drug. Option B is a Schedule II drug, and Option D is a Schedule I drug.

50. (C) They must have the same packaging.
This statement is false. For two drugs to be therapeutic equivalents, they must be approved by the FDA as effective and safe for use; meet standards of quality, strength, purity and identity; and be bioequivalent. They must be properly labeled and be manufactured according to the manufacturing guidelines. They can, however, differ in the way they are configured, shaped, scored, packaged and released and in the addition of excipients.

51. (C) Drugs with the same pharmacokinetics and pharmacodynamics.
Drugs with the same pharmacokinetics and pharmacodynamics best describe pharmaceutical equivalents. Option A describes bioequivalence. Option B describes pharmaceutical alternatives, and Option D describes therapeutic alternatives.

52. (B) Selectivity.
Selectivity is the extent to which a drug acts on a receptor site.

53. (A) Affinity.
Affinity is the probability of a drug occupying a receptor. The affinity of a drug to a receptor can be affected by both intracellular and external factors. Aging, genetic disorders and mutations can increase or decrease the affinity of receptors.

54. (B) Partial agonist.
Partial agonists have both agonist and antagonistic properties. They act as agonists when they are the only molecules bound to the receptors. However, when another agonist binds to the receptor, it becomes antagonistic. For example, pentazocine has agonistic effects on opioid receptors but becomes antagonistic if another opioid binds to the receptor.

55. (B) Water-soluble molecules diffuse quickly.

This statement is false about passive diffusion across membranes because molecules that are lipid soluble diffuse the fastest. Small molecules diffuse faster than large ones. Un-ionized molecules are typically soluble in lipids and thus diffuse faster than ionized ones.

56. (B) Lipids are transported by this means.
This statement is false because lipids are readily transported by passive diffusion and not facilitated diffusion. An example of a molecule transported via facilitated diffusion is glucose.

57. (B) Active transport.
Active transport requires an expenditure of energy. Transport can occur upward on a concentration gradient. This form of transport is useful for drugs in the form of endogenous substrates (vitamins), ions, amino acids and sugars.

58. (C) Food delays gastric emptying.
This is correct. Although the stomach has a large surface area, it has a thick mucosa and a short transit time, which can affect the rate of drug absorption. For these reasons, drug absorption occurs primarily in the small intestine. Food delays gastric emptying time, particularly foods rich in fat.

59. (D) It has a narrow therapeutic index.
Drugs with a narrow therapeutic index are considered high-alert medications, as small changes in the dose or blood concentration can cause adverse events. This group of medications carries an increased risk of causing harm to the patient if used in error.

60. (C) Nonsteroidal anti-inflammatory drugs (NSAIDs).
NSAIDs are not high-alert medications. High-alert medications are a class of drugs with a narrow therapeutic index. They may cause persistent adverse reactions if medication error occurs. Examples of high-alert medications are insulin, anticoagulants, narcotics and sedatives.

61. (D) An example is acetaminophen.

Acetaminophen is not an example of a high-alert medication. High-alert medications have a narrow therapeutic margin. Little changes in dosage or blood concentration can cause serious side effects, and adverse effects can be persistent, life-threatening and require hospitalization or critical care.

62. (D) Store insulin in the fridge.
Storing insulin in the fridge is not useful for preventing errors in the drug's administration. Strategies for reducing the occurrences of risk during insulin administration include implementing a check-and-balance system, where one CPhT prepares the drug and another reviews it; separating insulin vials from heparin vials during storage; spelling out all units and avoiding abbreviations.

63. (C) Phlebitis.
Hypertonic saline is often used to manage patients with edema and tissue fluid congestion because it causes the movement of fluids from the tissue space to the intravascular space. Side effects of hypertonic saline include phlebitis at the site of injection, hypovolemia, shock, osmotic demyelination syndrome and hypernatremia.

64. (A) Patient safety.
Patient safety is defined as the patient's ability to be free from errors or injuries caused by medical care. Practices and interventions that reduce the occurrence of preventable adverse effects greatly affect the patient's safety.

65. (B) Use commercially available premixes.
This is not useful for reducing the risk of errors when administering heparin. Errors peculiar to the administration of heparin include storing heparin vials side by side with insulin vials, ambiguous labels and use of multidose containers. Strategies for eliminating these errors include storing heparin vials away from insulin vials, using standardized concentrations and using single-dose containers.

66. (D) Diarrhea.
This is not a withdrawal symptom of benzodiazepines. Features of benzodiazepine withdrawal are tachycardia, tachypnea, hyperpyrexia and

seizures. Features of barbiturate withdrawal include restlessness, increasing anxiety, hyperreflexia, muscle weakness, delirium, seizures that can progress to status epilepticus, insomnia, visual and auditory hallucinations and death.

67. (B) Vaccine product–related reaction.
A vaccine product–related reaction is caused by the properties of the vaccine. For example, some patients can experience edema of the limbs after a DTP vaccine.

68. (D) Barcode.
A barcode reduces the risk of human errors. A barcode is a tool used to identify medications. This tool was created to ensure that the right drugs are given to the right patients in the right doses.

69. (B) Pastes contain a higher amount of solids than creams.
This is true. Pastes are compounded in the same manner as ointments and creams. They remain stable at body temperature and contain a higher amount of solids compared to creams. Pastes may or may not contain medication.

70. (D) They do not bring about systemic effects.
This is false about the production of gels. Depending on their formulation, gels may act on the surface of the skin alone to produce a local effect. They may also penetrate the skin, reaching its deeper layers or be absorbed through the skin, bringing about a systemic effect.

71. (C) They do not contain medication.
This statement is false about creams. Creams are usually compounded for topical use and are a combination of oil and water. They may or may not contain medication and are compounded in the same manner as ointments.

72. (A) Ointments are water-based products.
This is false concerning the formulation of ointments. Unlike creams, which are water-based, ointments are oil-based products. Insoluble powders may be used during their compounding, but they are first reduced to fine powders and

then added to a base using geometric dilution. The final product should be smooth and not contain any abrasive particles.

73. (C) A tablet mold.
Tablet molds are least useful for compounding ointments. They are used to form prepared powder mixtures into tablets. These molds are commonly made of metal with various sizes of plate cavities. After the cavities are filled, pressure is applied to force the formed tablets out of the cavity so they can dry. An ointment may be prepared on a glass slide or a mortar. It is handled with a spatula.

74. (B) Almond butter.
Suppositories are useful when a drug is to be delivered for local systemic effects. The three common bases used when compounding suppositories are glycerinated gelatin, polyethylene glycol and cocoa butter. While glycerinated gelatin is a water-miscible base, polyethylene glycol (carbowax) is water-soluble. Both bases are useful in producing rectal and vaginal suppositories. Cocoa butter (theobroma oil) is fat soluble and useful for rectal suppositories.

75. (C) Receptor affinity.
Receptor affinity affects the therapeutic effects of a drug. The rate and extent of distribution are determined by tissue binding, the extent of perfusion, permeability of membranes, regional pH, the type of partition between tissue and blood and tissue mass.

76. (B) Acidic drugs have large volumes of distribution.
This statement is false because acidic drugs have small volumes of distribution. They are bound to protein and stay in the circulation longer. Basic drugs, on the other hand, can have large volumes of distribution because they are used up by tissues.

77. (B) Basic drugs readily bind to adipose tissue.
This statement is false because basic drugs bind readily to lipoproteins and alpha-1-acid glycoproteins.

78. (C) Choroid plexus.
The choroid plexus is not a component of the blood-brain barrier. The blood-brain barrier is made of tightly packed endothelial cells on a tightly packed basement membrane that is covered by an astrocytic sheath. The endothelial cells are impermeable to water-soluble molecules.

79. (D) The drug's pH.
The pH does not affect a drug's rate of metabolism. It can, however, affect the drug's absorption from the gut.

80. (A) First order.
In first-order kinetics, the rate of metabolism is in proportion to the fraction of unmetabolized drugs left. In zero-order kinetics, the rate of metabolism is maximum, and a fixed amount of drug is metabolized per time.

81. (B) Oxidation.
The most common reaction occurring in Phase I metabolism is oxidation. Oxidation is done by the cytochrome P-450 (CYP450) enzymes.

82. (C) Glucuronidation.
The most common form of phase II reaction is glucuronidation. It occurs in the liver microsomes.

83. (A) Urine.
Drug metabolites are excreted primarily via the kidneys as urine because they are water-soluble and have a higher polarity.

84. (B) Acidifying the urine increases the rate of excretion of weak acids.
This statement is false because acidic urine reduces the rate at which weak acids are excreted and stimulates reabsorption. Therefore, alkalinizing the urine improves the rate of excretion of weak acids.

85. (D) Ibuprofen competes with aspirin for the COX-1 receptor.
Patients who are on acetylsalicylic acid (ASA) for coronary artery disease should avoid taking ibuprofen because it binds reversibly to COX-1 and

prevents the irreversible binding of ASA to COX-1 receptors. Because ASA is unable to bind to COX-1, it is unable to acetylate the serine molecule on the COX-1 protein. This failure stimulates the synthesis of thromboxane A2, a mediator that stimulates platelet aggregation and increases the risk of myocardial infarction in patients with coronary artery disease.

86. (D) It blocks the transport of serotonin into platelets.
NSAIDs should not be taken together with selective serotonin reuptake inhibitors (SSRIs) like citalopram, because their pharmacodynamic interactions increase the risk of gastrointestinal bleeding. NSAIDs bind to COX-1 and prevent platelet aggregation. SSRIs, on the other hand, block the transport of serotonin into platelets and thereby prevent platelet aggregation. These combined effects increase the risk of gastrointestinal bleeding.

87. (C) NSAID and ACEI.
This drug-drug interaction increases the risk of hypertension, not gastrointestinal bleeding. NSAIDs can inhibit the blood pressure–lowering effect of ACEIs. Since NSAIDs block prostaglandin synthesis and reduce perfusion in the glomerulus, they can trigger a reactive renin secretion, which can inhibit the action of ACEIs.

88. (B) Serotonin syndrome.
Concomitant use of SSRIs and triptans can increase the risk of serotonin syndrome.

89. (A) Fluoroquinolone and erythromycin.
Concomitant use of quinolones and macrolides or quinolones and citalopram can increase the risk of Torsade de Pointes.

90. (D) Citalopram.
Calcium supplements and antacids containing calcium carbonate can inhibit the absorption of bisphosphonates, levothyroxine, quinolones and tetracycline. They do so by forming complexes with them.

Test 2: Questions

1. All except which of the following drugs should not be co-administered with warfarin?
   A. Verapamil
   B. Ketoconazole
   C. Erythromycin
   D. Aspirin

2. All these should not be co-administered with an SSRI except?
   A. Theophylline
   B. Propranolol
   C. Clozapine
   D. None of the above

3. Which of the following is the mechanism of interaction between a PPI and clopidogrel?
   A. Formation of an unabsorbable complex in the gut
   B. Competitive antagonism
   C. Potentiation effect
   D. Inhibition of metabolism

4. PPIs will increase the bioavailability of all except which of the following drugs?
   A. Diazepam
   B. Citalopram
   C. Clopidogrel
   D. Venlafaxine

5. Which of the following dietary supplements will inhibit the therapeutic effect of cisplatin?
   A. Vitamin C
   B. Licorice
   C. Kava

D. Black cohosh

6. Iron tablets can be taken with which of the following fluids?

A. Milk
B. Orange juice
C. Kale smoothie
D. Coca-Cola

7. A patient on an MAOI should be careful in the consumption of all except which of the following foods?

A. Cheese
B. Salami
C. Yogurt
D. Oranges

8. Patients on cyclosporine, midazolam and psychotropics should be counseled on their consumption of grapes and grapefruit juice. Which of the following best describes the interaction of grapefruit on these drugs?

A. It blocks absorption.
B. It induces metabolism.
C. It inhibits metabolism.
D. It antagonizes drug receptors.

9. A patient on warfarin should be counseled on the moderate consumption of all except which of the following vegetables?

A. Carrots
B. Brussels sprouts
C. Spinach
D. Parsley

10. A patient on an antihypertensive should be counseled on the use of licorice. Licorice increases the risk of _______________.

A. Hyponatremia
B. Hyperkalemia
C. Hypokalemia
D. Hypocalcemia

11. Regarding barcode technology in medication, which of the following is true?

A. Barcode technology has been shown to reduce medication errors.
B. Barcode readers may not be able to properly capture the image and scan the barcode on certain objects.
C. Drug products that have more than one barcode may cause scanning difficulty.
D. All of the above.

12. Which of the following terms describes a storage device that contains a list of drug inventory that is dispensed electronically to ensure that drugs are given to patients in a controlled manner?

A. Automated medication dispensing device
B. Barcode medication administration
C. Automated dispensing cabinet device
D. Automated dispensing drug storage device

13. Which of the following is not an automated dispensing cabinet error?

A. Refill of medication bins with the wrong product
B. The patient's failure to adhere to the drug regimen
C. Selecting an incorrect drug from a multidrug bin
D. Nonadherence to safety steps

14. Which of the following is not a factor that contributes to medication error?

A. Calculation error
B. Improper use of leading and trailing zeros
C. Consistent labeling of drug products
D. Cluttered work environment

15. Jane Doe, a CPhT, mistook an abbreviation for milligrams while constituting a sedative medication for a patient. This resulted in a drug overdose. Which of the following abbreviations can be mistaken for milligrams?

A. HS
B. T I W
C. µg
D. U

16. Choose the correct option. Which of the following can cause a decimal point error?

A. .2 mg of Benadryl
B. 2.5 mg of Benadryl
C. 5 mg of Benadryl
D. 15 mg of Benadryl

17. The impact of medication error includes all but ____________.

A. Negative patient outcomes
B. Prolonged hospital stays and increases in health-care costs
C. Loss of trust in health-care professionals
D. Reduced hospital stay

18. Published medication error rates are underestimated for which of the following reasons?

A. Some errors go undetected.
B. Errors are usually identified and corrected before medication reaches the patient.
C. There is no efficient means of reporting medication errors.
D. Most medication errors are not fatal.

19. Which of the following is not a high-risk medication?

A. Vincristine
B. Potassium chloride injection
C. Fentanyl
D. Chloroquine

20. A CPhT receives oral orders from a prescriber. Which of the following safety tools must she use to avoid medication errors?

A. 3-way repeat-back patient safety tool
B. 2-way repeat-back patient safety tool
C. 4-way repeat-back patient safety tool
D. 1-way repeat-back patient safety tool

21. Suppositories can be used to deliver medication to all except which of the following organs?

A. Rectum
B. Urethra
C. Vagina
D. None of the above

22. Which of the following statements is false concerning capsule formation?

A. Capsule shells can be hard or soft.
B. Capsule shells are made of gelatinous materials.
C. A capsule is filled using a wide-bore syringe.
D. Pill tiles are necessary for capsule formation.

23. All except which of the following statements concerning capsule sizes is true?

A. The largest oral size suitable for patients is two.
B. Capsule sizes for oral administration range from number 5 to number 000.
C. Capsules with the number 000 are the largest.
D. The right size for a capsule is determined by trying different sizes and weighing.

24. All except which of the following are correct when compounding tablets?

A. It is useful when compounding potent drugs in small doses.
B. Tablet molds consist of pegboards and perforated plates.
C. A moistening agent consisting of water and alcohol is necessary when compounding powders.
D. A diluent is usually not required.

25. Which of the following is false concerning the production of powder forms of medications?
   A. It is used when drug solubility or stability is the concern.
   B. Light powders are usually placed on top of heavier ones when blending heavy and light powders.
   C. Powder dosage forms may be useful when powders are too bulky to be made into a capsule.
   D. None of the above.

26. Which of the following is false concerning beaker tongs?
   A. They're usually made of stainless steel.
   B. They can be used for beakers ranging from 50 mL to 2,000 mL in size.
   C. They usually possess only two jaws.
   D. They usually resemble ordinary ice tongs.

27. Which of the following equipment is not useful for measuring liquids?
   A. Syringes
   B. Pipettes
   C. Conical graduates
   D. None of the above

28. Which of the following options concerning medicine cups is false?
   A. They usually have a maximum capacity of 40 mL.
   B. They are used for administering oral medications.
   C. Accuracy is reduced when measuring fluids below 5 mL.
   D. They may be used to dispense liquid or dry medications.

29. Which of the following statements is correct about souffle cups?
1 – They are used for dispensing tablets, capsules and other solid forms of medication.
2 – They usually have calibrations in milliliters.
3 – They are produced in a single size only.
4 – They are usually produced using paper.

A. 1 and 3
B. 3 and 2
C. 1 and 4
D. 1 only

30. Insulin pens are used for administering insulin. Which of the following is true concerning this device?

A. All insulin pens are reusable.
B. Insulin pens are less accurate than a syringe when delivering insulin.
C. Insulin pens may possess memory features.
D. Insulin needles have similar lengths with different thicknesses.

31. Which organ of the endocrine system regulates body metabolism?

A. The thymus
B. The thyroid gland
C. The pancreas
D. The pineal gland

32. Patients are more prone to hyperglycemia in what form of diabetes mellitus?

A. Type I
B. Type II
C. Type III
D. Type IV

33. Which of the following is true concerning the Combat Methamphetamine Act?

A. It was designed to stop the illegal use of methamphetamine and cocaine.
B. Legal drugs used to produce methamphetamine must be kept behind the counter or in locked cases.
C. All pharmaceutical firms selling these legal drugs must be registered with the US attorney general.
D. All of the above.

34. The notification of the FDA of potentially harmful products is made by ________________.

A. The company that makes the product
B. The Centers for Disease Control and Prevention
C. During inspection
D. All of the above

35. The FDA is responsible for the recall of which of the following products?

A. Cosmetics
B. Household equipment
C. Cleaning supplies
D. None of the above

36. When returning controlled substances from Schedule II, which of the following steps should be taken?

A. DEA Form 222 must be used.
B. The return of these substances must be from one DEA registrant to another.
C. Substances must be properly labeled.
D. All of the above.

37. Which of the following defines a Class I drug recall?
   A. The recall of a drug that will cause severe adverse effects or death when there is use or exposure to patients
   B. The recall of a drug that has passed its expiration date
   C. The recall of a legend drug
   D. The recall of drugs that have only a placebo effect

38. Which of the following is an example of a Class I recall?
   A. Botulinum toxin contamination of honey
   B. Salmonella contamination of peanut butter
   C. Escherichia coli contamination of tomato paste
   D. All of the above

39. The FDA recalled a batch of potentially harmful drugs from the public. Which of the following is not a reason for a drug recall by the FDA?
   A. The discovery of harmful or dangerous drugs
   B. Improperly labeled and packaged drugs
   C. Drugs that contain ingredients not intended for use
   D. Drugs that cause somnolence

40. Convert 29/3 to a mixed fraction.
   A. 7 ⅔
   B. 9 ⅔
   C. 7 ⅓
   D. 8 ⅔

41. Convert 10 ⅘ to an improper fraction.
   A. 45/5
   B. 54/5
   C. 450/5
   D. 45/4

42. What is the lowest common denominator for 5/6 and 1/24?
   A. 4
   B. 6
   C. 12
   D. 24

43. What is the lowest common denominator for 3/8 and 3/4?
   A. 2
   B. 4
   C. 8
   D. 16

44. Add 2/3 and 2/3.
   A. 1⅓
   B. 2⅓
   C. 3⅔
   D. 1⅔

45. Add 1/12 and 5/24.
   A. 7/12
   B. 7/24
   C. 1/4
   D. 1/2

46. Multiply 2/5 by 9/10.
   A. 18/50
   B. 9/25
   C. 4/25
   D. 1/25

47. The Roman numeral M represents which of the following numbers?
   A. 10
   B. 100
   C. 1,000
   D. 50

48. Express 1,557 in Roman numerals.

   A. LDMVII
   B. MLDVII
   C. MXDVII
   D. MDLVII

49. Which of the following is an effect of cephalosporins on urine dipstick urinalysis?

   A. False-positive glycosuria
   B. False-positive hematuria
   C. False-positive bilirubinuria
   D. False-positive asthenuria

50. Which of the following is an effect of ranitidine in biochemical tests?

   A. False-positive hematuria
   B. False-positive results for amphetamines
   C. False-positive results for elevated INR
   D. False-positive results for hyperglycemia

51. Which of the following drugs can create false-positive results for opioids?

   A. Daptomycin
   B. Ranitidine
   C. Rifampin
   D. Acetaminophen

52. Which of the following can create false-positive results for hyperglycemia?

   A. Atenolol
   B. Rifampin
   C. Ranitidine
   D. Cefuroxime

53. Which of the following drug formulations is made by adding syrup into a powdered drug and then rolling the mixture into an oval or round shape?

A. Tablet
B. Plaster
C. Pill
D. Capsule

54. Which of the following drug formulations is suitable for the delivery of oral drugs with unpleasant tastes and odors?

A. Caplets
B. Capsules
C. Powders
D. Lozenges

55. Which of the following drug formulations has a high sucrose content?

A. Spirit
B. Solution
C. Syrup
D. Tincture

56. Which of the following drug formulations has alcohol as its primary solvent?

A. Spirit
B. Solution
C. Syrup
D. Tincture

57. Which of the following is false about the intradermal route of injection?

A. The angle of insertion is 15°.
B. It is commonly used for administering insulin.
C. The most commonly used site is the middle of the forearm.
D. The back can also be used.

58. The IM route of injection is suitable for administering all except __________.

A. Vesicant drugs
B. Drugs with large volumes
C. Drugs that need rapid absorption
D. Emulsions

59. S-T-A-R is an acronym used to prevent medication errors in a busy pharmacy. What does the acronym stand for?

A. Stop-think-act-review
B. Steady-takeover-act-review
C. Slow-think-act-revisit
D. Stop-think-act-revisit

60. The systematic evaluation of a process that enables prediction of severity of error at different points in the process is called ____________.

A. Root-cause analysis
B. Failure mode and effect analysis
C. Standardization analysis
D. Multiple-check analysis

61. Which of the following steps is not involved in the process of evaluation using FEMA?

A. Listing potential areas that may lead to failure at each stage
B. The description of the failure of the process and the root cause
C. Estimation of severity, likelihood of occurrence and probability of identifying the occurrence
D. Patient counseling

62. The multiple-check system includes all except ___________.

A. A pharmacist reviewing a physician order
B. A nurse inspecting the dose from the pharmacy
C. A patient asking questions before taking medication
D. A technician recommending a product that is a best seller at the pharmacy

63. PDSA is an acronym for ____________.

A. Plan-do-study-act
B. Prepare-direct-study-act
C. Plan-do-study-act
D. Plan-direct-study-act

64. Identify the option that is most likely to cause a wrong-dose error.

A. 10 mg
B. 0.5 mg
C. 10.0 U
D. 100 mg

65. James, a technician working in the unit-dose chart fill area, notices that Effexor XR (venlafaxine extended-release) 37.5 mg is mixed with venlafaxine immediate release in the same storage bin. Which of the following steps is appropriate for James to take?

A. Make no changes, as both medications are of the same strength.
B. Change the label to indicate both drugs are in the same bin.
C. Modify the stock shelf so each drug form can have its own section or bin.
D. None of the above.

66. An amoxicillin suspension available in 500 mg/5 mL concentration is ordered for a patient. The order reads: take 1 g TID x 10 days. What is the best way to write the label to avoid possible medication errors?

A. Take 1,000 mg three times a day for 10 days.
B. Take 1 g three times a day for 10 days with meals.
C. Take 10 mL three times a day for 10 days.
D. Take 5 mL three times a day for 10 days.

67. The purpose of the National Medication Error Reporting program includes all except which of the following?

A. Health workers sharing their experiences on medication errors
B. Improved patient safety
C. Education of health personnel to prevent future errors
D. A platform for patients to share experiences on adverse drug effects

68. Tom, a new technician undergoing on-the-job training after filling the drug bins, failed to rotate the stock. He puts all the new stock in the front containers of the stock area. What form of error can be caused by Tom's inability to rotate the stock?

A. Wrong-dose error
B. Compliance error
C. Deteriorated-drug error
D. Omission error

69. Which of the following statements is false concerning insulin syringes?

A. All insulin syringes come in a single size.
B. The scale of measurement on syringes is in milliliters and units.
C. Insulin syringes are not reusable.
D. Syringes are made from plastic.

70. Which of the following is false concerning spacer devices?

A. They can be used in place of an inhaler.
B. They should be washed in cold soapy water.
C. The devices should be cleaned with a towel and stored.
D. They increase the risk for oral thrush.

71. Which of the following is incorrect regarding calibrated droppers?

A. They are used to administer liquid medications.
B. They are usually calibrated in milliliters.
C. The maximum capacity of a dropper is usually 2 mL.
D. They are used for oral medications only.

72. Which of the following patient information is required on a patient's medication form?

A. Medication order
B. Name
C. Allergies
D. All of the above

73. Which of the following is correct about oral syringes?

A. They can be attached to a needle.
B. They are used to administer oral and parenteral medications.
C. All syringes come in a single size.
D. None of the above.

74. Which of the following is not a kind of syringe for administering parenteral medications?

A. A tuberculin syringe
B. An insulin syringe
C. An oral syringe
D. A multi-shot needle syringe

75. Which of the following is not a principle of the Bloodborne Pathogens Standard?

A. Standard precautions
B. Post-exposure follow-up
C. Recordkeeping
D. Workplace controls

76. All except which of the following sites are suitable for giving an IM injection to a one-month-old infant?

A. Gluteus maximus
B. Vastus lateralis
C. Deltoid
D. Quadriceps

77. The angle of insertion for the subcutaneous administration of epinephrine is ______________.

A. 15°
B. 45°
C. 90°
D. 60°

78. Which of the following is not an example of a therapeutic side effect?

A. Dexamethasone, a corticosteroid used to stimulate fetal lung maturity
B. Terazosin, an alpha 1 adrenergic receptor blocker used to treat benign prostatic hyperplasia and hyperhidrosis and diaphoresis
C. Sildenafil, originally designed for pulmonary hypertension and used to treat erectile dysfunction
D. Oxytocin, used to stimulate uterine contractions

79. Which of the following statements is false about temperature conditions for storing drugs?

A. Drugs stored at room temperature are stored at temperatures from 25°C to 30°C.
B. Drugs stored at cold temperatures are stored at temperatures from 2°C to 8°C.
C. Drugs in freeze storage are stored at temperatures from -20°C to -10°C.
D. High temperatures trigger oxidation, hydrolysis and photolysis.

80. Which of the following is not a strategy for storing drugs that are sensitive to light?

A. Storing them in amber-colored bottles
B. Wrapping the packages with aluminum foil
C. Storing them away from direct sunlight
D. Storing them in glass cubicles

81. Which of the following statements is false about the use of glass containers to package drugs?

A. They have an acidic surface.
B. They can cause the precipitation of crystals.
C. They allow radiation.
D. They are resistant to chemical changes.

82. Which of the following is not a disadvantage of using plastic as a packaging material?

A. It can leach into the drug.
B. It is permeable to moisture.
C. It allows drug migration into the environment.
D. It can trigger the precipitation of crystals.

83. Which of the following is the most significant disadvantage of using metal as a drug container?

A. Corrosion
B. Leaching
C. Photolysis
D. Precipitation

84. Which of the following precautions is used to reduce the risk of rubber containers leaching into drugs?

A. Coating them with polymers
B. Treating them with steam
C. Coating them with aluminum
D. Storing them away from direct sunlight

85. Which of the following chemical degradations is characterized by the loss of hydrogen ions and electrons?

A. Photolysis
B. Hydrolysis
C. Oxidation
D. Reduction

86. Which of the following drugs is most vulnerable to photolysis?

A. Epinephrine
B. Spironolactone
C. Sodium nitroprusside
D. Chlorpromazine

87. Which of the following is not an example of the chemical degradation of a drug?

A. Hydrolysis
B. Absorption
C. Oxidation
D. Photolysis

88. Which of the following statements is true concerning the effects of pH on the rate of drug degradation?

A. Solutions with a high pH are not oxidized easily.
B. Solutions with a low pH are not oxidized easily.
C. The pH of a drug has no effect on its rate of degradation.
D. Buffered aspirin solutions decompose faster than unbuffered ones.

89. Caffeine is added to procaine to improve the medication's stability. Which of the following best describes the effect of caffeine on procaine?

A. Acidification
B. Surfactant
C. Complex formation
D. Antioxidant

90. The time it takes for a drug to degrade to 90% of its initial strength if it is stored in ideal conditions is called ____________.

A. Half-life
B. Shelf life
C. Expiration date
D. Order of reaction

Test 2: Answers and Explanations

1. (D) Aspirin.
Aspirin is an antiplatelet that can be used with warfarin for anticoagulant therapy. Interactions of old-generation macrolide antibiotics, like clarithromycin and erythromycin, can inhibit cytochrome P450 3A4 and the metabolism of warfarin. This increases the risk of bleeding. Other inhibitors that should not be used with anticoagulants include verapamil (a calcium channel blocker), ketoconazole and fluconazole.

2. (D) None of the above.
SSRIs inhibit CYP2D6 and CYP1A2. They can increase the bioavailability of all these drugs and must not be co-administered with SSRIs.

3. (D) Inhibition of metabolism.
PPIs inhibit CYP2C19. This inhibits the conversion of the prodrug clopidogrel into its active metabolite. Concomitant use increases the risk of acute coronary syndrome in patients with coronary artery disease. PPIs increase the bioavailability of citalopram and the risk of QT prolongation. It increases the bioavailability of diazepam.

4. (C) Clopidogrel.
PPIs inhibit CYP2C19 and increase the bioavailability of a lot of drugs. However, the inhibition of the conversion of the prodrug clopidogrel into its active metabolite means that the bioavailability of clopidogrel is reduced.

5. (D) Black cohosh.
Cisplatin is an anticancer drug. Black cohosh is an herbal supplement used to treat post-menopausal symptoms. Black cohosh inhibits the action of cisplatin.

6. (B) Orange juice.
The citric acid in orange juice improves the absorption of iron tablets from the gut.

7. (D) Oranges.
Aged and fermented foods contain tyramine, a neurotransmitter. When eaten in significant amounts, they can interact with MAOIs and trigger a hypertensive crisis.

8. (C) It inhibits metabolism.
Grapefruit juice and grapes inhibit CYP3A4 and can increase the bioavailability of a good number of drugs to toxic levels. Some of the drugs affected are midazolam, felodipine, cyclosporine, most psychotropics, anticonvulsants and anticoagulants.

9. (A) Carrots.
Carrots will not inhibit warfarin's action. Vegetables that are high in vitamin K (kale, Brussel sprouts, spinach and parsley) can inhibit the action of warfarin.

10. (C) Hypokalemia.
Licorice contains glycyrrhizin, which can inhibit 11-beta-hydroxysteroid dehydrogenase and induce hypokalemia and hypernatremia. It can interfere with both antiarrhythmics and antihypertensives.

11. (D) All of the above.
Barcode technology has been shown to reduce the risk of medication errors. However, there are limitations to the use of this technology, as it may not capture images on certain objects, such as small vials or syringes. Drug products with more than one barcode may also be difficult to scan, making it important to know which barcode to scan.

12. (A) Automated medication dispensing device.
An automated medication dispensing device is a storage device that contains a list of drugs that are dispensed electronically to ensure they are given to patients in a controlled manner. Barcode medication administration is an automated inventory control system that makes use of barcodes to prevent errors in drug administration in hospitals.

13. (B) The patient's failure to adhere to the drug regimen.
A patient's failure to adhere to a drug regimen constitutes a medication error. Automated dispensing cabinet errors include refilling medication bins with a wrong product, nonadherence to safety steps and selecting incorrect medication from a multidrug bin.

14. (C) Consistent labeling of drug products.
This is not a factor that contributes to medication errors. Factors that contribute to medication errors include calculation errors, improper use of leading or trailing zeros, inconsistent labeling of drug products, a cluttered work environment, use of abbreviations, improper use of technology, unclear communication and human factors.

15. (C) µg.
The abbreviation µg for (microgram) can be mistaken for mg (milligram) and this can lead to an overdose of patient medication.

16. (A) .2 mg of Benadryl.
Decimal point errors cause miscalculations. A decimal point error occurs when a leading zero is not placed in front of a number that is less than 1.

17. (D) Reduced hospital stay.
Medication errors will not lead to a reduced hospital stay. The impact of medication errors on the patient is vast. It can lead to negative patient outcomes, prolonged hospital stays, an increase in the cost of care and a distrust in health-care professionals.

18. (A) Some errors go undetected.
Medication errors are preventable. Errors are reported based on incident reports or reported safety events. However, some errors go undetected. Cross-checking a prescription may be necessary to identify and correct medication errors before the drugs get to the patient.

19. (D) Chloroquine.

Chloroquine is not a high-risk medication. High-risk medications include chemotherapeutic agents like vincristine and methotrexate, potassium chloride injections, and opioids like fentanyl, apomorphine, morphine and hydrocodone. Others include hypoglycemic agents like insulin and neuromuscular blocking agents like pancuronium, cisatracurium, atracurium and succinylcholine.

20. (A) 3-way repeat-back patient safety tool.
The 3-way repeat-back patient safety tool is used when receiving oral orders from a prescriber. It involves writing down the order and reading it back to the prescriber to ensure clarity. The prescriber should acknowledge that the order is correct as it is read back.

21. (D) None of the above.
Suppositories can be used to deliver drugs to the rectal, urethral, nasal, vaginal and auricular cavities. Rectal suppositories are bullet shaped, while urethral suppositories are shaped like a pencil. Vaginal pessaries are globular or oviform in shape, while suppositories compounded for use in the ear are conical. Choosing the proper mold is important when compounding suppositories. These molds are made of different materials, including rubber, stainless steel, brass and plastic.

22. (C) A capsule is filled using a wide-bore syringe.
This is false concerning capsule formation. Empty capsules are filled with medication using the punch technique. The powder is compressed on a pill tile with a spatula, and the empty capsule body is pressed repeatedly into the powder until full. The capsule is then weighed to ensure an accurate dose.

23. (A) The largest oral size suitable for patients is 2.
This is false. For oral administration, capsule sizes range from a minimum of 5 to a maximum of 000. Number 0 is usually the largest size suitable for oral use by patients. The appropriate size for a capsule is determined by trying different sizes, weighing and choosing the best fit.

24. (D) A diluent is usually not required.

This is false. When compounding tablets, a diluent made of a mixture of lactose, sucrose and a moistening agent is used. The diluent is triturated with the active ingredients, then the alcohol and water mixture is added to make a paste.

25. (B) Light powders are usually placed on top of heavier ones when blending heavy and light powders.
This is false concerning the production of powder forms of medications. When heavy and light powders are to be combined, heavy powders should be placed on top of lighter ones and then blended. In cases where two or more powders are to be mixed, each powder should be separately crushed to the same particle size as the others before they are blended.

26. (C) They usually possess only two jaws.
This is false concerning beaker tongs. Beaker tongs are used for lifting beakers on and off hot plates and other surfaces in the laboratory. They resemble ordinary ice tongs but may possess either two or three jaws. They are used to handle beakers with a capacity of 50 mL to 2,000 mL.

27. (D) None of the above.
A pipette is used to measure liquids that are less than 1.5 mL in volume. Conical graduates have a wide top and a wider base and are usually calibrated in both metric and apothecary units. However, cylindrical graduates are generally more accurate than conical graduates. Their sizes range from 5 mL to above 1,000 mL. The smallest graduate available should be used to measure a particular volume of liquid.

28. (A) They usually have a maximum capacity of 40 mL.
This is false. Medicine cups are used for administering oral drugs, which may be in liquid or dry form. Usually, they have a capacity of 30 mL (1 fluid ounce) and are graduated in milliliters, teaspoons and ounces. They are less accurate when measurements are below 5 mL, so a more appropriate device should be used when smaller volumes are required.

29. (C) 1 and 4.

Souffle cups are paper cups similar to medicine cups. However, they are used to dispense solid forms of medications, such as capsules and tablets. Sizes may vary and are usually not calibrated. These cups are disposable after use and also have nonpharmaceutical uses.

30. (C) Insulin pens may possess memory features.
This is true. Insulin pens may possess memory features that recall the amount and timing of the previous insulin dose. There are two kinds of insulin pens: disposable pens, which allow for single use only and are discarded once the prefilled insulin cartridge is emptied, and reusable pens, which contain a replaceable cartridge. Once emptied, the cartridge is removed and a new one is installed.

31. (B) The thyroid gland.
The thyroid gland is a butterfly-shaped gland located below the larynx. It produces hormones that help regulate body metabolism. Hormones produced by the thyroid gland include thyroxine. The thymus, pancreas and pineal gland do not secrete hormones necessary to maintain body metabolism.

32. (A) Type I.
In type I diabetes mellitus, inadequate levels of insulin are secreted into the bloodstream. This is usually diagnosed in childhood, and patients require exogenous insulin administration to regulate blood glucose.

33. (D) All of the above.
The Combat Methamphetamine Act was formed in 2005 to stop the illegal use of cocaine and methamphetamine. It states that legal drugs used in the production of methamphetamines, such as ephedrine and pseudoephedrine, be placed behind the counter or in locked cases. All those selling these legal drugs must be registered with the US attorney general, and individuals are allowed only 9 grams per month per person of these drugs.

34. (D) All of the above.
Notification of the FDA of potentially harmful products is done in several ways. The company that manufactures the product can notify the FDA. The

FDA may be notified by the CDC. The FDA can discover harmful products on routine inspection or hear about harmful products over news and multimedia outlets.

35. (A) Cosmetics.
The FDA is responsible for the recall of food, drugs and cosmetics that are deemed unfit or unsafe for human consumption. Recalls can be made in cases of food contamination by microorganisms, defective medications with serious adverse effects and defective medical supplies.

36. (D) All of the above.
When returning controlled substances from Schedule II, DEA Form 222 must be used and the drug should be returned between one DEA registrant and another. All returned substances must be properly labeled, and the description, product names, size and manufacturer names must be properly identified.

37. (A) The recall of a drug that will cause severe adverse effects or deaths when there is use or exposure to patients.
The FDA describes a Class I recall as the recall of drugs that have serious adverse effects or death when they are used by or exposed to patients.

38. (D) All of the above.
Botulinum toxin contamination of honey, salmonella contamination of peanut butter and E. coli contamination of tomato paste are all examples of scenarios that will lead to an FDA Class I recall. This is because these food contaminants can cause potentially fatal infections.

39. (D) Drugs that cause somnolence.
This is not a reason for an FDA drug recall. The reasons for the recall of drugs include the discovery of drugs that are harmful or dangerous, improperly labeled, or packaging and drugs contain ingredients that are not intended for human use.

40. (B) 9 ⅔.

A mixed fraction has a whole number and a proper fraction. Three divides 29 nine times, with a remainder of two.

41. (B) 54/5.
$10\frac{4}{5} = (5 \times 10 + 4)/5 = 54/5$

42. (D) 24.
The lowest common denominator is the smallest whole number that can be divided by the denominators without a remainder. Twenty-four can be divided by each of the denominators without leaving a reminder.

43. (D) 16.
The lowest common denominator is the smallest whole number that can be divided by the denominators without a remainder. Sixteen can be divided by each of the denominators without leaving a reminder.

44. (A) $1\frac{1}{3}$.
The common denominator is 3.
$(2 + 2) / 3 = 4/3 = 1\frac{1}{3}$

45. (B) 7/24.
The common denominator is 24.
$(2+5)/24 = 7/24$

46. (B) 9/25.
$(2 \times 9)/(5 \times 10) = 18/50 = 9/25$

47. (C) 1,000.
The Roman numeral M represents 1,000.

48. (D) MDLVII.
1,000 = M
500 = D
50 = L
7 = VII

49. (A) False-positive glycosuria.
Cephalosporins can create false-positive glucose results in the urine (glycosuria).

50. (B) False-positive results for amphetamines.
Ranitidine and labetalol can create false-positive results for amphetamines.

51. (C) Rifampin.
Rifampin can create false-positive results for opioids.

52. (A) Atenolol.
Acetaminophen, albuterol, lisinopril and atenolol can cause false-positive results of serum hyperglycemia.

53. (C) Pill.
A pill is a single dose of a drug made by adding a syrup into a powdered drug and then rolling the mixture into an oval or round shape.

54. (B) Capsules.
A capsule is a medication contained in a gelatinous shell. Gelatin shells are used to enclose granules, liquids, powders or a combination of these. They are ideally used for drugs with unpleasant tastes or odors. Capsules also include sustained-release capsules. Such drugs should never be dissolved or crushed because doing so can affect their timed release.

55. (C) Syrup.
A syrup is a liquid drug formulation with a high amount of sucrose (such as ipecac syrup).

56. (D) Tincture.
A tincture is a drug form in which alcohol is the primary solvent (such as iodine tincture).

57. (B) It is commonly used for administering insulin.

This statement is false because the intradermal route is often used for allergy testing and tuberculin testing.

58. (D) Emulsions.
Emulsions are not given intramuscularly. They are for oral use.

59. (A) Stop-think-act-review.
The acronym S-T-A-R is used in the STAR safety tool when performing tasks that are critical to prevent medication errors. The acronym STAR stands for Stop, Think before you act, Act to complete the task and Review work that has been done.

60. (B) Failure mode and effects analysis.
The failure mode and effects analysis is a process that enables the prediction of the severity of error that can occur at different points in the process. It focuses on finding the flaws within a system that enable human errors. FEMA evaluates why and how the error occurred. A root-cause analysis is used to evaluate errors that cause a patient harm and assesses how these errors can be avoided in the future.

61. (D) Patient counseling.
Patient counseling should be done to help prevent errors that occur in outpatient settings and is not a step in FEMA. The steps involved in the process of evaluation include listing of potential areas that may lead to failure at each stage, description of failure of the process and the root cause, estimation of severity, the likelihood of occurrence and the probability of identifying the occurrence.

62. (D) A technician recommending a product that is a best seller at the pharmacy.
This is not part of the multiple-check system, which is designed to prevent medication errors. Steps include the pharmacist reviewing a physician's order, a nurse inspecting the dose from the pharmacy and a patient asking questions and examining the drug before taking it.

63. (A) Plan-do-study-act.
The PDSA is a safety tool used to prevent medication errors and improve medication safety. The acronym stands for Plan-Do-Study-Act. This cycle seeks to identify problems and generate ideas that are used to resolve the problem. This quality tool is helpful in testing changes on a minimum scale before implementation.

64. (C) 10.0 U.
This is most likely to cause a wrong-dose error as it contains a trailing zero and an abbreviation that can cause a common error. Trailing zeros can cause a tenfold increase in the dose of medication and lead to adverse outcomes. The abbreviation U, whose intended meaning is units, may also be mistaken for zero and lead to a drug overdose. All the other options are least likely to cause a wrong-dose error.

65. (C) Modify the stock shelf so each drug form can have its own section or bin.
The best step for the technician to take is to modify the stock shelf so each drug form can have its section or bin. This is necessary to prevent the administration of the wrong-dose form. Changing the label to indicate both drugs are in the same bin is improper, as different forms of the same medication should not be stored together.

66. (C) Take 10 mL three times a day for 10 days.
In the amoxicillin suspension, 500 mg = 5 mL.
1,000 mg = x mL
1,000 mg ÷ 500 mg = 2
2 x 5 mL = 10 mL of amoxicillin

67. (D) A platform for patients to share experiences on adverse drug effects.
The National Medication Error Reporting program provides a platform for health-care personnel to share their experiences to enhance patient safety. It also enhances educational efforts to prevent future medication errors.

68. (C) Deteriorated-drug error.

Failure to rotate the stock would cause a deteriorated drug error, as the older stock may expire and be dispensed beyond their expiration date. Compliance errors occur when patients fail to adhere to the drug regime. Omission error occurs when there is a failure of administration of a drug to an inpatient or a patient in a long-term care facility or when a patient fails to take a prescribed dose at the appropriate time.

69. (A) All insulin syringes come in a single size.
This statement is false. Syringes are available in three different sizes: 0.3 mL, 0.5 mL and 1 mL. The choice of a syringe is determined by the number of units of insulin a patient is required to take. Insulin syringes are made from plastic and should be disposed of after use to reduce the chances of infection.

70. (D) They increase the risk for oral thrush.
A spacer device is a hollow plastic tube used with an inhaler to enhance the delivery of medications to the airways. The inhaler is attached to one end of the spacer device, while the user breathes through the other end. A spacer device should be washed in warm soapy water and thoroughly air-dried. Using a spacer device reduces the risk of some side effects of medications, such as oral thrush from inhaled corticosteroids.

71. (D) They are used for oral medications only.
This statement is incorrect regarding calibrated droppers. Droppers are used to deliver small amounts of liquid medications, usually 1 mL or less. They can be used to deliver medicines to the mouth, ears or eyes and are calibrated in milliliters.

72. (D) All of the above.
A medication form contains a list of important details regarding the patient, including name, age, prescription order and any known drug allergies. This form is attached to the patient's drawer or tray. Each patient has a unique drawer or tray assigned to them that is refilled daily to meet their medication needs.

73. (D) None of the above.

Oral syringes are used to dispense liquid medications orally. They are usually not designed to hold a needle and so should not be used to administer parenteral medications. Syringes are available in 1 mL, 3 mL, 5 mL and 10 mL sizes.

74. (C) An oral syringe.
An oral syringe is not designed for parenteral use and should be used only to give medications by mouth. Multi-shot needle syringes, insulin syringes, tuberculin syringes, dental syringes, etc., are parenteral syringes used to administer subdermal and IM and IV injections.

75. (A) Standard precautions.
This is not a principle of the Bloodborne Pathogen Standard. The principles of the Bloodborne Pathogens Standard include exposure control plans, universal precautions, hepatitis B vaccination, post-exposure follow-up, hazard communication and training, recordkeeping, engineering and workplace controls and use of personal protective equipment.

76. (C) Deltoid.
The vastus lateralis, which is located in the anterolateral surface of the thigh, is the safest injection site for infants. It is part of the quadriceps muscle. The deltoid muscle is not an acceptable injection site for infants but is safe enough for older children.

77. (B) 45°.
The angle of insertion for subcutaneous epinephrine, medications and local anesthetics is 45° and 90° for heparin and insulin. The maximum volume of drugs to be administered via this route is 2 mL.

78. (D) Oxytocin, used to stimulate uterine contractions.
This is not a therapeutic side effect of oxytocin but a primary effect of oxytocin. Side effects are secondary effects caused by a drug. They can be adverse or therapeutic.

79. (D) High temperatures trigger oxidation, hydrolysis and photolysis.

This statement is false because high temperatures trigger oxidation, hydrolysis and reduction (not photolysis).

80. (D) Storing them in glass cubicles.
This statement is false. Storing them in glass cubicles doesn't reduce the risk of photolysis.

81. (A) They have an acidic surface.
This statement is false because glass has an alkaline surface.

82. (D) It can trigger the precipitation of crystals.
This statement is false because it is a side effect of glass, not plastic.

83. (A) Corrosion.
Metals can be used to store ointments, pastes, creams and emulsions. They can, however, precipitate or corrode the drug. To overcome these challenges, the interior part of the containers should be coated with polymers.

84. (B) Treating them with steam.
Rubber containers can leach into the drug. This challenge can be overcome by treating rubber stoppers with water or steam. Metals are treated with polymers to reduce the risk of corrosion.

85. (C) Oxidation.
Oxidation is characterized by a loss of hydrogen ions and a loss of electrons.
Some drugs readily affected by oxidation include:
Ethers – Diethyl ether
Thioethers – Chlorpromazine
Carboxylic acids – Fatty acids
Thiols – Dimercaprol (BAL)
Catechols – Catecholamines

86. (C) Sodium nitroprusside.
Sodium nitroprusside has a shelf life of four hours if exposed to light.

87. (B) Absorption.
This is a form of a drug's physical degradation, not chemical degradation.

88. (B) Solutions with a low pH are not oxidized easily.
This is true. Solutions with low pH are not oxidized easily. The pH of a solution can influence the rate of degradation of its compound. For example, a buffered aspirin solution is stable at a pH of 2.4, but if the pH increases about 10, it quickly decomposes. The pH of a solution also influences its rate of oxidation.

89. (C) Complex formation.
Solutions with complexes have a lower rate of oxidation and hydrolysis. For example, caffeine is used to form a complex with procaine to reduce the rate of hydrolysis.

90. (B) Shelf life.
The shelf life of a drug is the time it takes for a drug to degrade to 90% of its initial strength if it is stored in ideal conditions.

Test 3: Questions

1. Which of the following statements is a benefit of the lot number assigned to products?
   A. It enables manufacturers to perform quality control checks.
   B. It allows relevant entities to calculate expiration dates.
   C. It is important when corrections or recall information about a batch of products are to be issued.
   D. All of the above.

2. Which of the following is false regarding lot numbers?
   A. Lot numbers are not assigned by the FDA.
   B. Each drug in a batch has a unique lot number.
   C. Lot numbers are important when identifying counterfeit medications.
   D. It is the same as the drug's batch number.

3. Concerning expiration dates of medications, which of the following is false?
   A. Stability tests must be conducted by the manufacturer according to FDA guidelines before expiration dates are established.
   B. Storage conditions may alter the viability of a drug before its expiration date.
   C. The expiration dates of medications cannot be extended.
   D. The stability, efficacy and quality of medication are reduced beyond its date of expiration.

4. Potential risks associated with taking expired medication include all except which of the following?
   A. Toxic substances may be produced, which can cause harm.
   B. Efficacy may be reduced.
   C. Side effects from these drugs may be worse.
   D. None of the above.

5. Side effects associated with the use of misoprostol include all except which of the following?
   A. Abdominal pain
   B. Cardiac arrhythmia
   C. Polycythemia
   D. Myocardial infarction

6. All except which of the following are purposes of inventory management?
   A. Ensuring the least possible time is spent ordering medications
   B. Increasing the cost of ordering medications from wholesalers
   C. Reducing the number of times medications unexpectedly run out of stock
   D. Avoiding costs associated with damage or expiration of products

7. Which of the following has a rate of reaction that depends on the concentration of the drug?
   A. First-order reaction
   B. Zero-order reaction
   C. Second-order reaction
   D. Third-order reaction

8. Which of the following best describes a zero-order reaction?
   A. The rate of the reaction depends on the product of the two concentrations.
   B. The rate of change depends on the concentration of the drug.
   C. The rate of the reaction is constant and does not depend on the concentration of the reactants.
   D. None of the above.

9. Which of the following is the most common order of reaction?
   A. Zero-order reaction
   B. First-order reaction
   C. Second-order reaction
   D. Third-order reaction

10. All these have a narrow therapeutic index except?
   A. Warfarin
   B. Digoxin
   C. Amikacin
   D. Ciprofloxacin

11. Which of the following is not an example of a physical incompatibility?
   A. Immiscibility
   B. Insolubility
   C. Liquefaction
   D. Hydrolysis

12. All except which of the following mixtures are prone to liquefaction?
   A. Camphor
   B. Phenol
   C. Aspirin
   D. Zinc oxide

13. All except which of the following are examples of indiffusible solids?
   A. Calamine
   B. Acetylsalicylic acid
   C. Chalk
   D. Sodium chloride

14. What is the weight of a 68 lb. child in kilograms?
   A. 45 kg
   B. 34 kg
   C. 31 kg
   D. 30 kg

15. How many mL are in 10 tablespoons?
   A. 20 mL
   B. 15 mL
   C. 150 mL
   D. 250 mL

16. How many fluid ounces are in 500 mL?
    A. 100 fl. oz
    B. 16.7 fl. oz
    C. 20 fl. oz
    D. 250 fl. oz

17. Jake, while compounding an IV preparation of 40 mEq/L of potassium chloride in 0.9% of sodium chloride injection, notices that the potassium chloride injection looks cloudy before preparing the IV bag. Which of the following should Jake do to prevent a medication error?
    A. Proceed with compounding the IV, as potassium chloride injections always appear cloudy.
    B. Place the potassium chloride injection in warm water for five minutes.
    C. Inform the pharmacist that the potassium chloride injection is cloudy and proceed to inspect other potassium chloride vials in stock.
    D. Replace the potassium chloride injection with a new one.

18. Which of the following terms refers to a drug that cannot be dispensed to the public except on the order of a physician or any other licensed prescriber?
    A. Over-the-counter medication
    B. Legend drug
    C. Generic drug
    D. Brand name drug

19. Which of the following is not an element of a medication order?
    A. Generic drug name
    B. Patient name and hospital number
    C. Frequency and duration of administration
    D. The patient's sexual orientation

20. The pharmacy purchasing and inventory control process impacts the ability of the system to provide five basic rights to the patient. Which of the following is not a basic drug right?

A. Provision of the right drug
B. Provision of the drug to the right patient
C. Right route of administration
D. Right price of medication

21. A CPhT erroneously dispensed the wrong dose of digoxin to a patient. The patient suffered a cardiac arrest, which necessitated CPR, defibrillation and ICU management. The patient subsequently made a good recovery and was discharged home. According to the NCC MERP index for categorizing errors, what is the classification of the severity of harm?

A. Category I
B. Category H
C. Category A
D. Category D

22. Which of the following is a national program that monitors medication errors?

A. MedWatch
B. Pharm Alliance
C. Drug watch
D. Drug enforcement agency DEA

23. The pharmacy department can educate its staff on medication errors by ____________.

A. Using summaries of established errors published in staff newsletters
B. Educating the staff through educational programs on medication errors
C. Discussing medication error as part of a staff meeting
D. All of the above

24. Reporting medication errors should be ___________.

A. Voluntary
B. Mandatory
C. Informal
D. Formal

25. Which of the following is a form of dangerous abbreviation?

A. U
B. QD
C. QOD
D. All the above

26. Which of the following statements is false concerning drug utilization review?

A. It is a systematic review of how drugs are prescribed and used at the pharmacy
B. It enables the pharmacist and health-care provider to keep track of medication that is frequently prescribed.
C. It tracks side effects experienced by patients.
D. It only tracks cases of drug abuse.

27. Which of the following is false about a soluset?

A. It reduces the risk of fluid overload in the pediatric population.
B. 1 mL of fluid is delivered in approximately 60 drops.
C. It has a Y-site for the administration of drugs.
D. It does not include a rotatory Luer lock.

28. Which of the following medications can be administered through a transdermal patch?

A. Estrogen
B. Nicotine
C. Fentanyl
D. All of the above

29. All except which of the following are advantages of unit-dose packaging?

A. It reduces the incidence of medication errors.
B. It improves overall monitoring of drug use and drug control.
C. It saves time and cost for the pharmacy.
D. None of the above

30. Inhalers are used in the treatment of certain respiratory conditions. Which of the following statements is false concerning this device?

A. Inhalers should be stored at room temperature.
B. The wrong technique may result in medication wastage.
C. The mouthpiece and canister can be washed using water.
D. Oral thrush may be a side effect of the use.

31. Concerning nebulizers, which of the following statements is false?

A. They turn gaseous medicine into a mist.
B. They can be either battery run or electricity powered.
C. They are easier to use in young children.
D. They allow multiple medications to be delivered at once.

32. Which of the following is not an advantage of delivering insulin through an insulin pen?

A. It is portable, convenient and discreet.
B. It does not allow for any wastage of insulin.
C. It delivers highly accurate doses of insulin.
D. It is easy to use and saves time.

33. Which of the following statements is false concerning a volumetric infusion pump?

A. It may be used to administer small amounts of fluid.
B. It can be used to deliver large amounts of fluid.
C. It is incapable of delivering fluid at a continuous rate.
D. The fluid rate can be adjusted to very slow or very fast.

34. IV cannulas come in all except which of the following sizes?
   A. 12
   B. 14
   C. 22
   D. 20

35. Which of the following statements is false concerning a syringe pump?
   A. It can deliver large amounts of infusions.
   B. It may be able to infuse and withdraw fluids.
   C. It can be used for both medical and nonmedical purposes.
   D. It may be able to accommodate multiple syringes.

36. Which of the following is not an example of an automated dispensing cabinet?
   A. Pyxis
   B. Medselect
   C. RxStation
   D. None of the above

37. Which of the following is not required by the Joint Commission to be documented by a pharmacy in the case of a drug recall?
   A. A written official policy by the pharmacy on how it will handle recalled drug and medical supplies
   B. Date of notification of recall
   C. The number of medication that was affected by the recall
   D. The pharmacy's DEA number

38. A red receptacle is used in the disposal of _____________.
   A. Sharps
   B. Antibiotic ointment
   C. Chemotherapeutic agents
   D. IV solutions

39. Jake, a CPhT, wants to dispose of an expired batch of epinephrine. Which of the following waste receptacles should he use?

A. Red receptacle
B. Black receptacle
C. Yellow receptacle
D. Green receptacle

40. John, a CPhT, is notified of a recalled batch of nebulizers in stock. Which of the following steps is appropriate for a pharmacy to take after being notified of the recall of the nebulizers?

A. Have a written policy on how it will handle the recalled nebulizers.
B. Contact all patients who have received the recalled nebulizer.
C. Return the nebulizers to the manufacturer for proper disposal.
D. All of the above.

41. Which of the following explains the mechanism of action of sulfonylureas?

A. It inhibits hepatic and renal gluconeogenesis.
B. It stimulates release of endogenous insulin.
C. It stimulates the peroxisome proliferator–activated receptor-gamma nuclear receptor.
D. It slows down gastric emptying.

42. The CPhT supervisor is notified of a batch of recalled medication in stock in the pharmacy. He is required to identify this drug batch by the manufacturer's assigned number. Which of these numbers will make the recall of all the defective drugs possible?

A. Batch number
B. Lot number
C. Recall number
D. Index number

43. The FDA recalls a batch of aspirin due to an incorrect expiration date on the manufacturer bottle. What class of drug recall is this?

A. Class I
B. Class II recall
C. Class III recall
D. Class IV recall

44. Which of the following is an alpha-glucosidase inhibitor?

A. Tolbutamide
B. Miglitol
C. Vildagliptin
D. Pramlintide

45. Which of the following is not among the list of recalled drugs?

A. Fen-Phen
B. Diethylstilbestrol
C. Thalidomide
D. Vasopressin

46. You are to give 2 L of an infusion in four hours. What is the flow rate in mL/min?

A. 10
B. 8
C. 16
D. 25

47. You are to give 1 L of an infusion in five hours. If the drop factor is 10 gtt/mL, what is the drop rate for this infusion?

A. 50 gtt/min
B. 30 gtt/min
C. 33 gtt/min
D. 40 gtt/min

48. The drop rate of an IV set is 20 gtts/min. If the drop factor of the set is 10 gtt/mL, what is the flow rate in mL/hr?

A. 200
B. 60
C. 120
D. 240

49. 500 mL of Ringer's lactate runs for four hours at 200 gtt/hr. What is the drop factor?

A. 16 gtt/mL
B. 1.6 gtt/mL
C. 0.16 gtt/mL
D. 160 gtt/mL

50. 1 L of dextrose solution is infused in two hours. If the drop factor is 20 gtt/mL, what is the flow rate in gtt/min?

A. 16.7 gtt/min
B. 167 gtt/min
C. 1.67 gtt/min
D. 0.167 gtt/min

51. An infusion set has a drop factor of 15 gtt/mL. If the flow rate is 60gtt/min, what is the hourly flow rate?

A. 40 mL/hr
B. 60 mL/hr
C. 240 mL/hr
D. 480 mL/hr

52. You are to infuse 2 L of dextrose saline in two hours with an infusion set with a drop factor of 15 gtt/mL. What is the flow rate of this infusion?

A. 50 mL/min
B. 100 mL/min
C. 150 mL/min
D. 250 mL/min

53. A patient is being infused with 2 L of dextrose solution at a rate of 50 mL/hr. How much fluid is infused in 30 minutes?

A. 100 mL
B. 200 mL
C. 50 mL
D. 25 mL

54. You are to infuse 500 mL of fluids in 30 minutes with an infusion set of 15 gtt/mL. What is the flow rate in gtt/min?

A. 200 mL/min
B. 333 mL/min
C. 250 mL/min
D. 150 mL/min

55. Which of the following drug formulations is expressed in w/w?

A. Ointment
B. Elixir
C. Syrup
D. Tincture

56. Which of the following is expressed in milliequivalents?

A. Heparin
B. Insulin
C. Dextrose saline
D. Potassium chloride

57. How many mL are in 5 teaspoons?

A. 10 mL
B. 20 mL
C. 25 mL
D. 50 mL

58. How many mL are in 10 tablespoons?
   A. 100 mL
   B. 50 mL
   C. 150 mL
   D. 200 mL

59. Convert 78° C to Fahrenheit.
   A. 263°F
   B. 26.3°F
   C. 172.4°F
   D. 17.24°F

60. Convert 78°F to Celsius.
   A. 25.76°C
   B. 82.8°C
   C. 30.6°C
   D. 56.7°C

61. How many grains are in 15 dr?
   A. 50 gr
   B. 100 gr
   C. 900 gr
   D. 1000 gr

62. Which of the following is not a unit used in the apothecary system?
   A. Dram
   B. Ounces
   C. Grain
   D. Pints

63. How many pints are in four quarts?
   A. 8 pints
   B. 10 pints
   C. 20 pints
   D. 12 pints

64. How many quarts are in a gallon?
   A. 10 quarts
   B. 4 quarts
   C. 6 quarts
   D. 8 quarts

65. A pharmacist is performing a retrospective drug review on insulin. A retrospective drug utilization review addresses all except which of the following issues?
   A. Drug-drug interactions
   B. Incorrect drug dosage
   C. Drug-patient precautions
   D. Therapeutic duplication

66. Which of the following is incorrect concerning effective handwashing?
   A. Liquid soaps should be used instead of bar soaps.
   B. Running water should be used instead of water basins.
   C. Terry cloth towels should be used instead of paper towels.
   D. Hand sanitizers should contain at least 60% alcohol.

67. Which of the following forms is used to report stolen controlled substances?
   A. DEA Form 222
   B. DEA Form 41
   C. DEA Form 106
   D. DEA Form 221

68. A patient is having trouble getting her insurance to cover medication for her gastroesophageal reflux disease. She meets Tim, a pharmacist who shows her she can get Prilosec over the counter without prior authorization. This case depicts which of the following?
   A. Therapeutic substitution
   B. Therapeutic intervention
   C. Therapeutic index
   D. Drug-drug substitution

69. John is a 54-year-old male on pain management for bone cancer. While checking his database, it is noticed that he gets refills of his opioid painkillers simultaneously from different pharmacies. Which of the following lines of action is most appropriate?

A. Report this to the FDA MedWatch.
B. Report the event to the drug enforcement agency DEA.
C. Talk it over with John and his health-care provider.
D. Ignore the event, as John is in a lot of pain.

70. Which of the following is not a purpose for drug utilization review?

A. To identify trends in prescribing among a group of patients
B. To enhance collaboration among the health-care team to improve drug therapy among patients
C. To emphasize the need for therapeutic substitution and legend drugs
D. To foster efficient utilization of health-care resources

71. Which of the following forms is used to return damaged controlled substances?

A. DEA Form 222
B. DEA Form 41
C. DEA Form 106
D. DEA Form 221

72. A patient reports a history of allergic reactions when she takes sulfur-containing medication. Allergic reactions to medication include all except which of the following?

A. Hives
B. Wheezing
C. Cough
D. Shortness of breath

73. Jane has been having flu-like symptoms for the past three days. She buys an over-the-counter flu medication. Where can she find the side effects of the medication?

A. Ask her partner, who has taken the medication before.
B. Check the label.
C. Ask a forum on an online website.
D. Book an appointment to ask her health provider.

74. Which over-the-counter medication has a warning label that it can potentially cause liver damage?

A. Aspirin
B. Warfarin
C. Acetaminophen
D. Heparin

75. How many drams are in 5 fluid ounces?

A. 20 drams
B. 100 drams
C. 50 drams
D. 40 drams

76. Convert 5 mg to micrograms.

A. 5,000 mcg
B. 500 mcg
C. 0.005 mcg
D. 50,000 mcg

77. Convert 5 pt to fl. oz.

A. 80 fl. oz
B. 50 fl. oz
C. 25 fl. oz
D. 10 fl. oz

78. Which of the following is the mechanism of action of clonidine?

A. Angiotensin-converting enzyme inhibitor
B. Calcium channel blocker
C. Alpha-adrenergic agonist
D. Beta-blocker

79. All except which of the following antihypertensives are unsuitable for use in pregnancy?

A. Methyldopa
B. Lisinopril
C. Telmisartan
D. Spironolactone

80. Which of the following antihypertensives may be unsuitable for a patient with uncontrolled diabetes?

A. Lisinopril
B. Propranolol
C. Telmisartan
D. Nifedipine

81. All except which of the following are significant side effects of sublingual nitroglycerin?

A. Postural hypotension
B. Reflex tachycardia
C. Rebound hypertension
D. Peripheral edema

82. Concerning nitroglycerin, which of the following statements is false?

A. It reduces preload.
B. It should not be combined with sildenafil.
C. It shouldn't be used as monotherapy.
D. It is a vasodilator.

83. Which of the following drugs inhibits platelet aggregation?

A. Warfarin
B. Dabigatran
C. Triflusal
D. Streptokinase

84. Which of the following drug pairs have similar therapeutic effects?

A. Warfarin and streptokinase
B. Aspirin and dabigatran
C. Triflusal and clopidogrel
D. Heparin and alteplase

85. Which of the following drugs has an oral form?

A. Dabigatran
B. Alteplase
C. Heparin
D. Streptokinase

86. Which of the following is not a Class Ia antiarrhythmic drug?

A. Disopyramide
B. Lidocaine
C. Quinidine
D. Procainamide

87. All except which of the following are side effects of Class II antiarrhythmics?

A. Hyperglycemia
B. Hypotension
C. Bradycardia
D. Urinary retention

88. Which of the following describes the mechanism of action of Class III antiarrhythmics?

A. Sodium channel blockers
B. Beta-blockers
C. Potassium channel blockers
D. Calcium channel blockers

89. All except which of the following are side effects of Class IV antiarrhythmics?

A. Rashes
B. Photodermatitis
C. Peripheral edema
D. Constipation

90. All except which of the following are examples of Class V antiarrhythmics?

A. Phenytoin
B. Magnesium sulfate
C. Digoxin
D. Adenosine

Test 3: Answers and Explanations

1. (D) All of the above.
In addition to the options listed, a lot number also provides an identifier that a consumer can use to contact the manufacturer of a product or to research the production of goods received.

2. (B) Each drug in a batch has a unique lot number.
A lot (batch) number is a unique number assigned to a particular batch of products from a single manufacturer, not individual drugs. The batch of medicines produced at the same time is assigned the same lot number. This number is not assigned by the FDA but by the manufacturer of the product.

3. (C) The expiration dates of medications cannot be extended.
The expiration date of a drug may be extended by the manufacturer based on testing and acceptable data per the protocol approved in the new drug application (NDA) or abbreviated new drug application.

4. (D) None of the above.
There are several risks associated with taking medications that are expired or have been poorly stored. Such drugs might have reduced efficacy because their strength has been lowered. Toxic substances may also be yielded from these drugs, which can cause serious side effects. Persons with life-threatening and serious diseases are more susceptible to these potential risks.

5. (C) Polycythemia.
Polycythemia is not a side effect of misoprostol. Misoprostol is a synthetic prostaglandin E analog that inhibits the synthesis of prostaglandins, inhibits gastric acid secretion and protects the gastric mucosa. It also binds to myometrial cells, causing strong myometrial contractions. Side effects include diarrhea and abdominal pain, cardiac arrhythmias, myocardial infarction and anemia.

6. (B) Increasing the cost of ordering medications from wholesalers.

This is not a purpose of inventory management. Proper inventory management ensures that medications do not run out unexpectedly, the cost of ordering medications from wholesalers is reduced, minimal time is spent ordering and purchasing medications, and costs associated with expired or damaged goods are prevented.

7. (A) First-order reaction.
A first-order reaction is the most common reaction. Here the rate of change depends on the concentration of the drug.

8. (C) The rate of the reaction is constant and does not depend on the concentration of the reactants.

9. (B) First-order reaction.
A first-order reaction is the most common reaction. Here the rate of change depends on the concentration of the drug.

10. (D) Ciprofloxacin.
Ciprofloxacin has a wide therapeutic index. Drugs with a wide therapeutic index include B-lactams, quinolones and macrolides.

11. (D) Hydrolysis.
This is a form of chemical (not physical) incompatibility

12. (D) Zinc oxide.
Zinc is not prone to liquefaction. Some mixtures are eutectic because their melting point is reduced until it is below room temperature. Hydrates are then released. It is difficult to compound such mixtures because they are liquid. Examples include menthol, camphor, phenol, aspirin, chloral hydrate and sodium salicylate.

13. (D) Sodium chloride.
Sodium chloride is not an indiffusible solid. Common examples of indiffusible solids are zinc oxide, chalk, succinylsulfathiazole, calamine and acetylsalicylic acid.

14. (C) 31 kg.
To convert pounds to kilograms, divide by 2.2.
68 lbs/2.2 = 30.9 kg = 31 k

15. (C) 150 mL.
1 tablespoon = 15 mL
10 tablespoons = 150 mL.

16. (B) 16.7 fl. oz.
1 fluid ounce = 30 mL
X = 500 mL
X = 16.67 oz = 16.7 fl. oz

17. (C) Inform the pharmacist that the potassium chloride injection is cloudy and proceed to inspect other potassium chloride vials in stock.
Potassium chloride injections come as a clear liquid, and cloudiness may be an indication of an expired or poorly stored batch of medication. Jake should inform the pharmacist if clear suspensions or injections appear cloudy and proceed to inspect other batches to confirm if the stock is expired.

18. (B) Legend drug.
Legend drugs are medications that cannot be dispensed to the public unless on the order of a physician or other licensed prescriber. They are also called prescription drugs. An OTC medication does not require a prescription to be sold to the public and should be properly labeled for home use.

19. (D) The patient's sexual orientation.
A patient's sexual orientation is not an element of a medication order. A medication order is a written request on a physician's order form or a transcribed verbal order in an inpatient setting. The elements of a medication order include the drug's generic name, brand name if applicable, frequency and dose of administration, route of admission, strength, dosage form, indication for use of medication, prescriber's signature and credentials, date and time of order.

20. (D) Right price of medication.
Right price of medication is not a basic drug right. The pharmacy purchasing and inventory control process enables the provision of the right drug to the right patient, in the right amount, in the right dosage form, by the right route of administration and at the right time and frequency.

21. (B) Category H.
According to the NCC MERP index of categorizing medical errors, the case scenario described is a Category H medication error. In Category H, an error occurs that requires a life-sustaining treatment, such as CPR, defibrillation and intubation. Category I medication error may have contributed to or resulted in the death of a patient. Category A includes circumstances that can cause an error, and Category D includes errors that reached the patient and required monitoring to confirm they caused no harm to the patient.

22. (A) MedWatch.
MedWatch is a national program by the FDA that monitors medication errors. The FDA MedWatch, the Institute of Safe Medication Practice (ISMP) and Medication Error Reporting Program (MERP) monitor medication errors and issues concerning the integrity of products and confusing labels. The DEA oversees drug trafficking and drug distribution.

23. (D) All of the above.
The pharmacy department can educate staff on medication errors by using summaries of established errors published in staff newsletters, educating the staff through educational programs on medication errors and discussion of medication errors as part of a staff meeting.

24. (A) Voluntary.
Medication errors should be reported whenever they occur. However, this process is voluntary. Medication error reporting programs include the FDA MedWatch program and the ISMP medication error reporting program. Reporting of medication errors is not mandatory, required by state law or illegal.

25. (D) All the above.
The use of error-prone or dangerous abbreviations—such as U for units, QD for every day and QOD for four times daily—should be discouraged, as medication errors occur when prescribers use these abbreviations.

26. (D) It only tracks cases of drug abuse.
This is false. The drug utilization review is a systematic review of how drugs are prescribed and used at a pharmacy. It enables the pharmacist and health provider to keep track of frequently prescribed patient medications, therapeutic effects, side effects and success rates of medications.

27. (D) It does not include a rotatory Luer lock.
This is false. A soluset (Buretrol) is used to administer fluids in the pediatric population. It consists of a graduated burette that possesses inlets for air and fluids and also has a filter at its base. A tube delivers fluid from the burette to the patient and may have a Y-site through which IV medications can be administered. A rotatory Luer lock secures the tube to the IV cannula.

28. (D) All of the above.
A transdermal patch delivers medications topically from where they are absorbed into the bloodstream. Estrogen, nicotine and fentanyl can all be administered through a transdermal patch. These patches allow for small amounts of drugs to be delivered into the bloodstream over a long period. The amount of drug a patch delivers and the length of time it needs to be worn varies among patches.

29. (C) It saves time and cost for the pharmacy.
This is not an advantage of unit-dose packaging. A unit-dose system of distributing medication allows for a pharmacy-controlled method of dispensing and controlling medications. It is especially beneficial in preventing errors associated with medication dispensing and may save costs for patients. However, it requires more pharmacy processing time and equipment cost.

30. (C) The mouthpiece and canister can be washed using water.
This is false. To keep an inhaler clean, the mouthpiece and cap can be rinsed in warm water and allowed to air dry. No other parts should be rinsed, such as the canister. Inhalers are used to deliver medication in gaseous form into the airways. If used incorrectly, they may result in wastage of medication and increase the chances of oral thrush, as the medicine may remain in the oral cavity and not reach the respiratory system.

31. (A) They turn gaseous medicine into a mist.
This is false. Nebulizers turn liquid medications into a mist, allowing them to be absorbed into the lungs. They require a battery or an electricity source to be used and are easier to use in young children, as all the children need to do is inhale and exhale. Nebulizers can be used to deliver multiple medications at once. However, not all respiratory medications can be given through a nebulizer.

32. (B) It does not allow for any wastage of insulin.
Insulin pens are easy to use, especially for children and older adults, and save time during use, as the insulin levels are already prefilled and preset. They also have the advantage of being portable and allowing the user to be discreet during administration. However, a small amount of insulin is wasted with each use.

33. (C) It is incapable of delivering fluid at a continuous rate.
This is false. Volumetric pumps are capable of delivering specific amounts of infusions, and infusion rates can be adjusted from very slow to very fast to suit the patient's needs. They are used commonly to control the flow rate of IV medications, fluids, blood and blood products and to deliver fluids at a continuous flow rate.

34. (A) 12.
IV cannulas are used to secure IV access, which is necessary when a medication or fluid is to be given through the vein. These cannulas come in different sizes, ranging from 14G to 26G, with 14G being the largest and 26G

being the smallest. Cannulas are color coded. IV cannulas do not come in size 12.

35. (A) It can deliver large amounts of infusions.
This is false. Syringe pumps (syringe drivers) are used to deliver fluids in small amounts, with or without medication, to patients. There are different kinds of syringe pumps, and they can be used for both medical and industrial purposes. They are designed to deliver fluids at a predetermined speed and rate.

36. (D) None of the above.
Automated dispensing cabinets facilitate the administration of patients' medications. Examples include Pyxis, Medselect and RxStation

37. (D) The pharmacy's DEA number.
The pharmacy's DEA number does not need to be documented in case of a drug recall. The Joint Commission requirements on documentation of drug recall by a pharmacy include a written official policy by the pharmacy on how it will handle recalled drugs and medical supplies, the date the pharmacy was notified of recalls, the number of medications affected by the recall, the number of patients affected by the recall and a detailed description of the action that was taken with regards to recalled medication.

38. (A) Sharps.
The red receptacle bin is used in the disposal of sharps, such as needles, syringes and materials that contain bodily fluids and blood (IV catheters). It is made of thick plastic material to prevent these objects from poking out. Chemotherapeutic agents are disposed of in the yellow receptacle. All IV solutions that do not contain medication should be disposed of in the water drain. The blue receptacle is used to dispose of expired antibiotic ointment and noncontrolled drugs, like aspirin.

39. (B) Black receptacle.
The black receptacle is used to dispose of medications that are controlled and hazardous, such as epinephrine and chemotherapeutic agents. A red

receptacle is used in the disposal of sharps, such as needles and syringes that have been contaminated with bodily fluids and are potentially infectious. The red sharps bin is made with thick plastic material and is puncture proof. The yellow receptacle is used in the disposal of potentially toxic and hazardous materials to the environment, such as chemotherapeutic agents.

40. (D) All of the above.
The recall of defective medical supplies, such as nebulizers, would require the pharmacy to have a written policy on how to handle recalled nebulizers, contact all patients who have received the recalled nebulizers and return these recalled nebulizers to the manufacturer for proper disposal.

41. (B) It stimulates release of endogenous insulin.
Insulin secretagogues stimulate the release of endogenous insulin by facilitating the closure of K+ channels in the beta cells. Examples include sulfonylureas like tolbutamide, second-generation sulfonylureas (glimepiride), glipizide and glyburide. Others include repaglinide, nateglinide and meglitinide.

42. (B) Lot number.
The lot number is a number the manufacturer assigns to individual drugs to enable the pharmacy to identify drugs that have been recalled. Batch number, index number and recall number are incorrect answers.

43. (C) Class III recall.
Recall of an aspirin batch due to the incorrect expiration date is an example of a Class III drug recall. A Class III recall is the recall of a drug wherein its use or exposure is not likely to cause any adverse health consequences.

44. (B) Miglitol.
Alpha-glucosidase inhibitors inhibit alpha-glucosidase, an enzyme responsible for converting complex sugars to monosaccharides. This action reduces postprandial hyperglycemia. Examples are miglitol and acarbose.

45. (D) Vasopressin.

Vasopressin is not a drug that has been recalled. Fen-Phen, diethylstilbestrol and thalidomide are among the list of drugs recalled in the United States. Fen-Phen, a drug combination of fenfluramine and phentermine used to combat obesity, was recalled due to pulmonary hypertension and rare valvular heart defects seen in patients on this medication. Diethylstilbestrol was recalled due to vaginal and uterine anomalies in the daughters of women exposed to it. Thalidomide, which was used to prevent nausea and vomiting in pregnancy, was recalled as it caused phocomelia in the fetus.

46. (B) 8.
Flow rate = volume/time
Volume in mL = 2,000 mL
Time in minutes = 240 minutes
2,000 mL/240 minutes = 8.33 = 8 mL/min

47. (C) 33 gtt/min.
Drops per minute = [Total IV volume/Time (minute)] X Drop Factor

Drops per minute = ?
IV volume = 1L = 1,000 mL
Time = 5 hours = 300 minutes
Drop Factor = 10 gtt/mL

Drops per minute = (1,000 mL/300 minutes)
× 10 gtt/mL
Drops per minute = 33.33 gtt/min = 33 gtt/min

48. (C) 120.
Drops per minute = [Total IV volume/Time (minute)] X Drop Factor

Drops per minute = 20 gtts/min
Drop factor = 10 gtt/mL
Flow rate = Y
20 gtts/min = Y × 10 gtt/mL
Y = 20 gtts/min/10 gtt/mL

Y = 2 mL/min

Convert mL/min to mL/hr
2mL / 1 = X/60 minutes
X = 120 mL/hr

49. (B) 1.6 gtt/mL.
Find the flow rate in mL/hr. Then use it to divide the flow rate in gtt/hr.

Flow rate in mL/hr = 500 mL/4 hours = 125 mL/hr
200 gtt/hr/125 mL/hr = 1.6 gtt/mL.

50. (B) 167 gtt/min.
Drops per minute = [Total IV volume/Time (minute)] X Drop Factor

Drops per minute = ?
Drop factor = 20 gtt/mL
V = 1L = 1,000 mL
Time = 2 hours = 120 minutes.

Drop per minute = (1,000 mL/120 minutes) × 20 gtt/min
Drop per minute = 8.33 mL/minute × 20 gtt/min
Drop per minute = 166.6 gtt/min = 167 gtt/min

51. (C) 240 mL/hr.
Drops per minute = [Total IV volume/Time (minute)] X Drop Factor

Drops per minute = 60 gtt/min
Drop factor = 15 gtt/mL
V =?
Time =?

60 gtt/min = (flow rate) × 15 gtt/mL
Flow rate = 60 gtt/min/15 gtt/mL
Flow rate = 4 mL/min

Convert to hours = 240 mL/hr

52. (D) 250 mL/min.
Drops per minute = [Total IV volume/Time (minute)] X Drop Factor

Drops per minute = X
Drop factor = 15 gtt/mL
V = 2 L = 2,000 mL
Time = 2 hours = 120 minutes

X = (2,000 mL/120 minutes) × 15 gtt/mL
X = (16.67 mL/min) × 15 gtt/mL
X = 250.05 mL/min
X = 250 mL/min

53. (D) 25 mL.
50 mL/hr × 1 hr/60 mins × 30 minutes = 25 mL

54. (B) 333 mL/min.
Drops per minute = [Total IV volume/Time (minute)] X Drop Factor

Drops per minute = X
Drop factor = 15 gtt/mL
V = 500 mL
Time = 30 minutes

X = (500 mL/30 minutes) × 15 gtt/mL
X = (16.67 mL/min) × 30 gtt/mL
X = 333 mL/min

55. (A) Ointment.
Percentage w/w is the number of grams in 100 grams of a solution. It is in %w/w. It is used to measure powdered substances prepared with semisolid or solid substances, like ointments, pastes and creams.

56. (D) Potassium chloride.
A milliequivalent is used to measure the number of protons in a liter of salt solutions, like potassium chloride.

57. (C) 25 mL.
1 teaspoon = 5 mL
5 teaspoons = 25 mL

58. (C) 150 mL.
1 tablespoon = 15 mL
10 tablespoons = 150 mL

59. (C) 172.4°F.
°F = °C × (9/5) + 32
°F = 78°C × 1.8 + 32
°F = 172.4°F

60. (A) 25.76°C.
°C = (°F – 32) × (5/9)
°C = (78°F -32) × (0.56)
°C = 46 × 0.56
° C = 25.76°C

61. (C) 900 gr.
1 dr = 60 gr
15 dr = 900 gr

62. (D) Pints.
The apothecary system is not common in the United States. It is an old system of measurement. It is also called the US liquid measure system and the wine measure system. Weight is measured in grain (gr), dram and ounces (and not pints).

63. (A) 8 pints.
1 quart = 2 pints

4 quarts = 8 pints

64. (B) 4 quarts.
1 gallon = 4 quarts

65. (C) Drug-patient precautions.
A retrospective drug utilization reviews drug therapy after a patient has received medication. It addresses issues such as drug-drug interactions, incorrect drug dosage, therapeutic duplication, clinical drug misuse or abuse, inappropriate duration of drug treatment and incorrect utilization of drugs. This type of review does not address drug-patient precautions.

66. (C) Terry cloth towels should be used instead of paper towels.
This statement is incorrect because disposable paper towels should be used instead of cloth towels.

67. (C) DEA Form 106.
As soon as a controlled substance is noted to be lost or stolen, the nearest DEA office must be promptly contacted and notified using DEA Form 106. The notification report must include the name of the company and its address, the date the item was lost or stolen, the pharmacist's DEA number, a list of all missing drugs and costs of purchase and an update from the local police.

68. (A) Therapeutic substitution.
Therapeutic substitution occurs when an already prescribed drug is replaced with an alternative medication that is assumed equal in the therapeutic effect.

69. (C) Talk it over with John and his health-care provider.
Opioid medications are frequently misused and have a high tendency for addiction. Any suspected case of drug misuse should be talked over by the patient and prescriber to prevent adverse outcomes.

70. (C) To emphasize the need for therapeutic substitution and legend drugs.
This is not a purpose of drug utilization review. Drug utilization review helps to identify trends in prescribing among a group of patients, enhance

collaboration among the health-care team to improve drug therapy among patients and foster efficient utilization of health-care resources.

71. (B) DEA Form 41.
DEA Form 41 is used to report damaged and outdated controlled substances. The pharmacist will also attach a cover letter that describes the state of the drugs and request permission to destroy them. Retail pharmacies can make this request once a year.

72. (C) Cough.
A cough is not an example of an allergic reaction. Allergic reactions to medication are caused by hypersensitivity. Symptoms of allergic reactions include hives, wheezing, shortness of breath, itching, fever, rashes, swelling and anaphylactic shock in severe cases. Different patients have varying degrees of sensitivity to the same medication.

73. (B) Check the label.
The side effects of medications can be found on the drug label. The patient can read the drug label to learn about the side effects. Care must be taken to label medication properly. Incorrect labeling of drugs is an indication of a drug recall.

74. (C) Acetaminophen.
Acetaminophen has a warning on the drug label of its potential to cause liver damage. Caution should be taken when dosing this readily available OTC medication.

75. (D) 40 drams.
1 fluid ounce = 8 drams
5 fluid ounces = 40 drams

76. (A) 5,000 mcg.
1 mg = 1,000 mcg
5 mg = 5,000 mcg

77. (A) 80 fl. oz.
1 pt = 16 fl. oz
5 pt = 80 fl. oz

78. (C) Alpha-adrenergic agonist.
This class of drug stimulates alpha 2 adrenergic receptors in the brain stem and reduces the activity of the sympathetic nervous system. Side effects include depression, drowsiness and lethargy. Examples include clonidine, methyldopa and guanfacine.

79. (A) Methyldopa.
The following drugs are suitable for pregnancy because of their low risk for teratogenicity: alpha agonists (methyldopa), hydralazine, calcium channel blockers and beta-blockers.

80. (B) Propranolol.
Propranolol is a beta-blocker that reduces heart rate without reducing cardiac output. A significant adverse effect of this drug is hyperglycemia. This side effect makes this drug unsuitable in a patient with uncontrolled diabetes.

81. (D) Peripheral edema.
Peripheral edema is a side effect of calcium channel blockers, not nitroglycerin.

82. (A) It reduces preload.
This statement is false because nitroglycerin reduces afterload (peripheral vascular resistance).

83. (C) Triflusal.
Triflusal is a COX-2 inhibitor. It binds to the serine residue on COX-2 and irreversibly inhibits the action of COX-2 in initiating platelet aggregation.

84. (C) Triflusal and clopidogrel.
Triflusal is a COX-2 inhibitor, while clopidogrel is an ADP inhibitor. Both drugs inhibit platelet aggregation.

85. (A) Dabigatran.
Dabigatran is an anticoagulant that inhibits Factor IIa. It is available orally. The other medications listed are given subcutaneously and intravenously because they must bypass the gut.

86. (B) Lidocaine.
Lidocaine is a Class Ib (not Class Ia) antiarrhythmic drug.

87. (D) Urinary retention.
Urinary retention is a side effect of sodium channel blockers (Class I). Class II antiarrhythmics are beta-blockers. Side effects include bradycardia, hypotension, hypoglycemia, hyperglycemia, difficulty breathing (bronchoconstriction), depression, dizziness and fatigue.

88. (C) Potassium channel blockers.
Class III antiarrhythmics are potassium channel blockers. Examples include sotalol, amiodarone, bretylium, betapace and dronedarone.

89. (B) Photodermatitis.
Photodermatitis is a side effect of potassium channel blockers (Class III). Class IV antiarrhythmics are calcium channel blockers. Examples are verapamil, diltiazem and isoptin. Side effects include constipation, hypotension, edema, nausea, rashes and headaches.

90. (A) Phenytoin.
Phenytoin is a Class Ib (not Class V) antiarrhythmic drug.

Test 4: Questions

1. Which of the following is false concerning perpetual inventory systems?
   A. Federal law requires its use for all medications.
   B. It is used to record the amount of a particular medication available in a pharmacy.
   C. It is managed through a computerized system.
   D. Medications that fall below the reorder points can be automatically reordered.

2. Barcodes can be useful for all except which of the following in a pharmacy setting?
   A. To verify prescriptions before they are issued
   B. To ensure correct medications are given at the right time
   C. To create labels for a patient's prescription vial
   D. To increase the chances of errors in dispensing

3. Which of the following external factors will not affect the availability of a medication to be ordered?
   A. Drug recalls
   B. Decreased availability of raw materials
   C. Higher than usual demands
   D. The pharmacy's purchasing power

4. Which of the following statements about the turnover rate of products is false?
   A. Turnover rate may be affected by a pharmacy's location.
   B. The turnover rate may change at different times of the year.
   C. Drugs with low turnover rates should be kept at maximum stock levels.
   D. The turnover rate refers to how fast medication is used up.

5. When receiving controlled substances, which of the following is untrue?
   A. It should be verified that the package has not been tampered with.
   B. They can be shipped together with other medications.
   C. Pharmacists must receive controlled substances once they arrive.
   D. Controlled substances must be stored differently.

6. Which of the following is untrue about receiving and handling investigational drugs?
   A. Policies and procedures for handling these drugs are not necessary.
   B. Invoices for these drugs must be kept separately.
   C. They can be received similarly to other medications.
   D. Pharmacies may require logbooks for receiving and dispensing these drugs.

7. Which of the following is not a potassium-losing diuretic?
   A. Torasemide
   B. Eplerenone
   C. Hydrochlorothiazide
   D. Ethacrynic acid

8. Which of the following diuretics increases the risk of gynecomastia?
   A. Torasemide
   B. Eplerenone
   C. Hydrochlorothiazide
   D. Ethacrynic acid

9. Which of the following is a selective COX-2 inhibitor?
   A. Sulindac
   B. Acetaminophen
   C. Celecoxib
   D. Naproxen

10. An NSAID like ibuprofen increases the risk of gastrointestinal bleeding because of its effects on prostaglandin synthesis in the mucosa lining of the stomach. Which of the following enzymes is responsible for the synthesis of prostaglandin?

A. Thromboxane
B. COX-1
C. COX-2
D. Phospholipase A2

11. Which of the following best describes the mechanism of action of acetaminophen?

A. COX-1 inhibitor
B. COX-2 inhibitor
C. CNS suppression
D. Thromboxane inhibitor

12. All except which of the following are symptoms of opioid withdrawal?

A. Diarrhea
B. Rhinorrhea
C. Pinpoint pupils
D. Fever

13. All except which of the following anticonvulsants work by blocking sodium channels?

A. Phenytoin
B. Lamotrigine
C. Carbamazepine
D. Ethosuximide

14. Ms. Gracie is on a prescription for phenobarbital for a seizure disorder. Which of the following describes the mechanism of action of phenobarbital in controlling the seizures?

A. GABA enhancer
B. Sodium channel blocker
C. Calcium channel blocker
D. NMDA receptor agonist

15. A 14-year-old female who is taking an antiseizure drug has hyperplasia of her gums. Which of the following drugs is implicated?

A. Ethosuximide
B. Phenytoin
C. Diazepam
D. Levetiracetam

16. All except which of the following are typical effects of anticonvulsants?

A. Teratogenicity
B. Liver enzyme induction
C. Allergic reactions
D. Anemia

17. Which of the following terms defines a patient's ability to take prescription medication correctly?

A. Medication adherence
B. Medication avoidance
C. Medication attentiveness
D. Medication aversion

18. Which of the following does not improve medication adherence?

A. Polypharmacy
B. Patient education on the importance of medication adherence
C. Modification of the patient's beliefs and human behavior
D. Family support

19. The acronym SIMPLE is used in which of the following strategies?
   A. Drug adherence intervention strategy
   B. Drug substitution strategy
   C. Drug adverse effect limitation strategy
   D. Drug abuse prevention strategies

20. Which of the following is not a means of evaluation adherence to drug regimen?
   A. Use of PHQ-9
   B. Use of Morisky-4 scale
   C. Review medication containers and refill dates
   D. Asking about adherence behavior in every visit

21. Why was Baycol, a brand name for cerivastatin, recalled?
   A. Teratogenicity
   B. Rhabdomyolysis
   C. Pulmonary fibrosis
   D. Phocomelia

22. Barriers to medication adherence include which of the following?
   A. The patient's misconstrued perception of the disease
   B. Inadequate insurance coverage
   C. Frequent treatment changes and adjustment
   D. All of the above

23. Which of the following is not a health system–related factor in poor drug adherence?
   A. Poor insurance coverage
   B. Inadequate time with the health-care provider
   C. Poor patient follow-up
   D. Side effects of the medication

24. Concerning separating inventory, which of the following is false?

A. Medications with similar names or packaging should be stored in the same location.
B. The inventory should be limited to prevent overcrowding.
C. Adequate lighting should be maintained.
D. Medication should be kept at eye level with labels facing outward.

25. Lola, a 44-year-old female, presents to her general practitioner with eczema. Her practitioner prescribes a topical steroid. He fills out the prescription and writes, "Apply hydrocortisone lotion 1.0% on the affected area TID for 5 days." What medication error can Lola's physician's prescription result in?

A. Wrong-dose error
B. Wrong-route-of-administration error
C. Deteriorated-drug error
D. Omission error

26. A CPhT and his colleagues are having issues deciphering a prescription. Which of the following steps is most appropriate?

A. Reject the prescription.
B. Type in the best possible interpretation of the drug prescription.
C. Call the primary care physician for clarification.
D. Advise the patient on an OTC medication to take.

27. Which of the following is false about a modified unit dose?

A. It is also known as a blister card.
B. It is also known as a blended unit dose.
C. It packages medications sufficient for one month into a card.
D. It is a kind of unit-dose system.

28. Which of the following orders is incorrectly matched?
   A. Admitting order – Contains previous medications taken and new medications being ordered
   B. STAT order – Contains medications needed immediately or for an emergency
   C. PRN order – Given at the same time daily, based on physician's direction
   D. Discharge order – Medicines patients should continue to take upon discharge until they can follow up with their physician

29. A urethral catheter can be made from all except which of the following materials?
   A. Latex
   B. Silicone
   C. Polyurethane
   D. Rubber

30. Which of the following color codes for IV cannulas is incorrectly matched?
   A. 14G – Orange
   B. 18G – Pink
   C. 24G – Yellow
   D. 16G – Gray

31. Which of the following is true about the National Drug Code (NDC)?
   A. It is unique for every new drug produced.
   B. It is reviewed every 20 years.
   C. It is the same as the national formulary.
   D. The name of each drug is included in its code.

32. All except which of the following information is supplied by the NDC?
   A. Manufacturer or distributor of the drug
   B. Drug formulation
   C. Size of its packaging
   D. Color of the medication

33. Which of the following is likely to be an NDC number for a medication?
   A. NDC 0071-62
   B. NCD 7759- 002-35
   C. NDC 03261-559-28
   D. NCD 6652-74-32-87

34. Which of the following statements is correct concerning the national drug number?
   A. Drugs are never removed from the NDC list.
   B. The NDC number is usually a 10-digit code.
   C. It is the same as the prescription number.
   D. Drug codes for different drugs may be swapped based on the manufacturer's discretion.

35. Which of the following measuring conversions is false?
   A. 1 g = 1 cc of water
   B. 1 g = 15 gr
   C. 1 g = 0.034 oz
   D. 1 g = 1,000 mcg

36. Which of the following is not an example of an automated dispensing cabinet?
   A. Pyxis
   B. Medselect
   C. RxStation
   D. None of the above

37. Which of the following best describes a Class II drug recall?
   A. Recall of a drug that will cause serious adverse effects or death when used
   B. Recall of a drug or violative product that can cause reversible health consequences
   C. Recall of a drug unlikely to cause any adverse health effects
   D. Recall of a drug with has a high cost

38. Which of the following is not a criterion used to identify hazardous drugs?

A. Carcinogenicity
B. Teratogenicity
C. Organ toxicity at high dose
D. Genotoxicity

39. Personal protective equipment worn when handling hazardous materials includes all except _____________.

A. Safety boots
B. Respirators
C. Face shields
D. Powdered gloves

40. Which of the following statements is false about the use of PPE in compounding areas for hazardous drugs?

A. Head, hair and shoe covers reduce the chances of microbial or particulate contamination in areas where hazardous drugs are compounded.
B. Wearing head, hair and shoe covers outside compounding areas may put unprotected workers at risk.
C. Head, hair and shoe covers may protect workers from the residues of hazardous materials on floors and other contact areas.
D. None of the above.

41. Which of the following statements is untrue about respirators?

A. Respirators protect against gases and vapors.
B. Respirators do not offer much protection against liquid splashes.
C. A NIOSH-certified N95 mask may be used.
D. Respirators offer protection against airborne particles.

42. Which of the following does not apply to gloves used for personal protection?
   A. Powder-free gloves should be used.
   B. Gloves should be inspected for physical defects before use.
   C. Gloves with long cuffs should be placed under the cuff of the gown.
   D. Two pairs of gloves should be worn.

43. Which of the following is untrue regarding gowns worn as PPE?
   A. It is recommended that gowns be changed every three hours during extended work with hazardous substances.
   B. Gowns that have been tested to resist permeability by hazardous materials should be worn.
   C. Surgical scrubs and cloth laboratory coats are ideal outerwear when handling hazardous drugs.
   D. Gowns should close at the back and not have an open front.

44. All except which of the following items can be used for eye and face protection when handling hazardous substances?
   A. Face shields
   B. Goggles
   C. Full facepiece respirators
   D. None of the above

45. Which of the following is not a component of a spill kit used during exposure to hazardous drugs?
   A. First aid box
   B. Waste containers
   C. Absorbent pads
   D. Deactivating agents

46. Concerning accidental exposure, which of the following is true?
   A. All workers involved with hazardous substances have a potential for accidental exposure.
   B. The material safety data sheet (MSDS) contains information about potential hazards associated with materials.
   C. Filing an incident report is relevant only for large-scale exposures.
   D. Spill kits are important in facilities utilizing hard drugs.

47. Express 2571 in Roman numerals.
   A. MMDLXXI
   B. MMDLVII
   C. MMDVIII
   D. MLDLXXI

48. A prescription order is as follows: 500 mg Metformin bid for 14 days. The drug available is Glucophage 250 mg/tablet. How many tablets will be dispensed?
   A. 70
   B. 56
   C. 46
   D. 28

49. A physician's order is as follows: Ampicillin 0.5 g, PO, tid for 7 days. The available drug is ampicillin 250 mg. How many capsules will be dispensed?
   A. 24
   B. 42
   C. 48
   D. 28

50. The physician's prescription is as follows: Acetaminophen 500 mg PO qid. The dose on hand is 250 mg/5 mL. How many mL will be dispensed?
   A. 5
   B. 10
   C. 0.5
   D. 1

51. The prescription order is as follows: Heparin 10,000 units SC. The available dose is 40,000 units/mL. How many mL will be administered?

A. 1
B. 1.25
C. 0.25
D. 1.5

52. A prescription order requests that 50,000 units of a drug be added to an IV solution. The available dose is 10,000 units/1.5 mL. How many mL will be used?

A. 5.5
B. 7.5
C. 7
D. 8.5

53. A prescription order is as follows: Gentamicin 60 mg IM tid for 7 days. The available strength is 80 mg/2 mL ampoule. How many ampoules will be used?

A. 20
B. 16
C. 18
D. 10

54. The prescription order is as follows: Atropine 0.2 mg SC stat. The available dose of atropine is 0.4 mg/mL. How many mL will be given to this patient?

A. 1
B. 0.5
C. 0.2
D. 1.5

55. A physician's order is as follows: Heparin 7,500 units SC. The available dose is 10,000 units/mL. How many mL will be given?

A. 7.5
B. 2.5
C. 0.75
D. 0.25

56. Milo is on a prescription of phenelzine, diazepam, acetaminophen and carbamazepine. He comes to the pharmacy with dyspnea, breathlessness and palpitations. On examination, his blood pressure is 150/110 mmHg. His face is also flushed. There is a history of consumption of gruyere cheese and salami at a garden party. Which of the following drugs is most implicated?

A. Phenelzine
B. Diazepam
C. Acetaminophen
D. Carbamazepine

57. Which of the following pairings has a synergistic effect?

A. Levodopa and amantadine
B. Levodopa and carbidopa
C. Levodopa and pramipexole
D. Levodopa and selegiline

58. All except which of the following are side effects of levodopa?

A. Dyskinesia
B. Hyperprolactinemia
C. Psychosis
D. Postural hypotension

59. Which of the following drugs is a dopamine receptor agonist?

A. Bromocriptine
B. Pramipexole
C. Levodopa
D. Biperiden

60. Which of the following is not a first-generation antipsychotic?

A. Haloperidol
B. fluphenazine
C. Thioridazine
D. Clozapine

61. Which of the following is false about second-generation antipsychotics?
   A. They have a high affinity for D2 receptors.
   B. They have a lesser risk for extrapyramidal effects.
   C. They block 5-HT2 receptors.
   D. They block alpha-adrenergic receptors.

62. Which of the following is an effect of the blockade of 5-HT2 receptors?
   A. Galactorrhea
   B. Low libido
   C. Sedation
   D. Postural hypotension

63. Marcus is a 45-year-old male on olanzapine. He complains of delayed ejaculation. Which of the following best describes the mechanism of action of this occurrence?
   A. M receptor blockade
   B. Alpha-adrenergic receptor blockade
   C. 5-HT2 receptor blockade
   D. D2 receptor blockade

64. All except which of the following effects are likely with a first-generation antipsychotic?
   A. Tardive dyskinesia
   B. Neuroleptic malignant syndrome
   C. Low libido
   D. Postural hypotension

65. A patient has a prescription for imipramine. What class of drug is this?
   A. SSRI
   B. SNRI
   C. MAOI
   D. TCA

66. A CPhT receives a prescription order and dispenses the drug accordingly. During the dispensing process of medication, what is the first step in which a medication error can be prevented?

A. Filling in a prescription
B. Patient consultation
C. Recording the prescription
D. Labeling

67. The process by which medications prescribed for a patient by a medical practitioner are checked to ensure that they match the current list of drugs that a patient is taking is referred to as ______________.

A. Medication review
B. Medication reconciliation
C. Medication cross-check
D. Medication management

68. What is the aim of medication reconciliation used by health facilities?

A. To reduce the cost of medication
B. To improve the therapeutic effect of medication
C. To avoid medication errors
D. To enhance facilitation of the transfer of care

69. All except ____________ are pharmacokinetic properties of drugs.

A. Drug absorption
B. Drug distribution
C. Drug excretion
D. Drug half-life

70. Severe unwanted symptoms that develop due to the administration of a drug are called _____________.

A. Side effects
B. Adverse effects
C. Idiosyncratic reaction
D. Hypersensitivity reaction

71. A unique, unpredicted and strange reaction to a drug is called _____________.

A. Idiosyncratic reaction
B. Adverse reaction
C. Hypersensitivity reaction
D. Side effects

72. Hypersensitivity reaction has been linked to all except which of the following drugs?

A. Penicillin
B. Sulfamethoxazole
C. Aspirin
D. Niacinamide

73. Concerning an anaphylactic drug reaction, which of the following is true?

A. It is a severe form of an allergic reaction.
B. It constitutes a medical emergency.
C. Respiratory paralysis can occur.
D. All of the above.

74. The interference of a drug with the effect of another drug, nutrient or laboratory test is called _____________.

A. Drug interaction
B. Drug reaction
C. Drug action
D. Drug metabolism

75. The cooperative effect of two or more drugs given together that produces a stronger effect than when either of the drugs is given alone is called _____________.

A. Potentiation
B. Synergism
C. Antagonism
D. Additive effect

76. Which of the following is an example of a serotonin 5-HT2 antagonist?

A. Phenelzine
B. Mirtazapine
C. Trazodone
D. Bupropion

77. John is a 27-year-old male on citalopram. He should be counseled on the causes of serotonin syndrome. Which of the following interactions does not increase the risk of serotonin syndrome?

A. Meperidine
B. Dextromethorphan
C. St John's wort
D. Ibuprofen

78. Which of the following is not a direct-acting cholinergic?

A. Pilocarpine
B. Neostigmine
C. Carbachol
D. Nicotine

79. Which of the following is false about organophosphates?

A. They are long-acting inhibitors of acetylcholinesterase.
B. Malathion is an example.
C. They can be used to treat myasthenia gravis.
D. They work on both muscarinic and nicotinic receptors.

80. Which of the following direct-acting agonists stimulates both nicotinic and muscarinic receptors?

A. Nicotine
B. Pilocarpine
C. Varenicline
D. Carbachol

81. All except which of the following are features of parasympathetic stimulation?

A. Mydriasis
B. Diarrhea
C. Bronchoconstriction
D. Micturition

82. All except which of the following are signs of atropine toxicity?

A. Tachycardia
B. Xerostomia
C. Hyperthermia
D. Diaphoresis

83. Charlie is on a prescription of scopolamine for seasickness during his boat cruise. All except which of the following are expected side effects of this drug?

A. Sedation
B. Urinary urgency
C. Constipation
D. Flushing

84. Which of the following acts on both alpha and beta-adrenergic receptors?

A. Clonidine
B. Dobutamine
C. Phenylephrine
D. Norepinephrine

85. Which of the following is a physiological response of stimulation of alpha-adrenergic receptors?

A. Tachycardia
B. Miosis
C. Bronchoconstriction
D. Vasodilation

86. Which of the following adrenergic drugs is the drug of choice for anaphylaxis?

A. Dobutamine
B. Dopamine
C. Phenylephrine
D. Epinephrine

87. All except which of the following beta 2 adrenergic agonists are suitable for prophylaxis of asthma?

A. Albuterol
B. Formoterol
C. Olodaterol
D. Salmeterol

88. Which of the following drugs is suitable for causing mydriasis without causing cycloplegia?

A. Atropine
B. Tropicamide
C. Phenylephrine
D. Albuterol

89. Which of the following adrenergic drugs is suitable for use in an obstetric patient experiencing uterine cramps in the first trimester?

A. Salbutamol
B. Phenylephrine
C. Dobutamine
D. Clonidine

90. An obstetric patient is on a prescription of terbutaline for premature labor. Which of the following is a likely effect of this drug?

A. Hyperglycemia
B. Tachycardia
C. Bronchoconstriction
D. Hepatitis

Test 4: Answers and Explanations

1. (A) Federal law requires its use for all medications.
This is false. Federal law requires the use of perpetual inventory systems for Schedule II controlled substances (although they are also required to be managed on paper as well). While it is not a federal requirement, using this system for all medications ensures that an accurate stock of medications is always reflected in the pharmacy's computer system. Where reorder points or periodic automatic replacement levels are set, medications can be automatically reordered by the system to replace medications that are below the set mark.

2. (D) To increase the chances of errors in dispensing.
Barcodes do not increase the chances of errors in dispensing. Barcode technology has actually significantly reduced the occurrence of errors during pharmaceutical processes. Using barcodes, medications can be verified before they are issued. It can also ensure that the correct medication is used to fill a prescription and given to patients at each point in time.

3. (D) The pharmacy's purchasing power.
The availability of certain medications can be affected by external factors, including issues with the manufacturing process, decreased availability of raw materials to compound the product and higher-than-normal demand for the medication. The pharmacy's purchasing power is not an external factor affecting the availability of the drug, as other pharmacies with more funds at their disposal will be able to purchase the drug if the manufacturer makes it available.

4. (C) Drugs with low turnover rates should be kept at maximum stock levels.
This is false. Medications with low turnover should be kept at minimum stock. Turnover rate refers to the time it takes to use up a particular medication in the pharmacy's inventory. Some drugs have a high turnover rate, and technicians should ensure those drugs are always available to fill prescriptions.

5. (B) They can be shipped together with other medications.
This is untrue. Controlled substances are drugs or chemicals whose manufacture, use or possession are controlled by the government. These products should be shipped separately from other products, and it is necessary to verify that the package has not been tampered with before it is opened. The CPhT must hand over these substances to the pharmacist upon receipt.

6. (A) Policies and procedures for handling these drugs are not necessary.
This is untrue. Policies and procedures are required to handle these drugs.

7. (B) Eplerenone.
This is an aldosterone antagonist that prevents the excretion of potassium and reabsorption of sodium in the distal and collecting tubules. It is a potassium-sparing diuretic.

8. (B) Eplerenone.
This drug is an aldosterone antagonist. It blocks the action of aldosterone and prevents the excretion of potassium and reabsorption of sodium in the distal and collecting tubules. Side effects include polyuria, diarrhea, stomach cramps, hyperkalemia and gynecomastia.

9. (C) Celecoxib.
This is a selective COX-2 inhibitor with minimal risk for gastrointestinal bleeding and kidney disease. Other examples include Firocoxib, parecoxib and lumiracoxib. Sulindac and naproxen are nonselective COX-2 inhibitors, while acetaminophen has no anti-inflammatory effect.

10. (B) COX-1.
Cyclo-oxygenase 1 (COX-1) is colloquially known as the housekeeping enzyme. It is responsible for cell signaling and cytoprotection (synthesis of prostaglandins required for coating the stomach mucosa). Nonselective COX inhibitors like ibuprofen block the action of this enzyme and increase the risk for gastrointestinal ulcers.

11. (C) CNS suppression.
Acetaminophen has no inflammatory properties since it does not inhibit COX. It works directly in the brain by inhibiting the transmission of pain signals to thalamic and cortical centers.

12. (C) Pinpoint pupils.
Pinpoint pupils are symptoms of opioid overdose. Symptoms of opioid withdrawal include anxiety, tachypnea, diaphoresis, lacrimation, yawning, rhinorrhea, diarrhea, anorexia, tremors, fever, tachycardia, hypertension and stomach cramps. Symptoms are usually not fatal. Overdose symptoms include respiratory depression, apnea, miosis, hypotension, delirium, bradycardia, hypothermia and urinary retention.

13. (D) Ethosuximide.
Ethosuximide is a calcium channel blocker, not a sodium channel blocker. Other examples of calcium channel blockers are ethosuximide, gabapentin, pregabalin and valproic acid.

14. (A) GABA enhancer.
Barbiturates stimulate GABA secretion by binding to receptors located on chloride ion channels. By binding to them, they keep chloride ion channels open for longer. They also work by blocking glutamate receptors.

15. (B) Phenytoin.
Side effects of phenytoin include gingival hyperplasia, hirsutism, peripheral neuropathy, nystagmus and induction of hepatic enzymes.

16. (D) Anemia.
Anemia is not a typical effect of anticonvulsants. Typical effects include allergic reactions, like Stevens-Johnson syndrome, skin rashes, teratogenicity, induction of liver enzymes and CNS effects.

17. (A) Medication adherence.
Medication adherence is a patient's ability to take prescribed medication correctly. It involves taking the correct medication at the right dosage and at

the right time, as well as getting refills in a timely manner. Various factors affect drug adherence (lack of finances and poor communication between patients and the health team).

18. (A) Polypharmacy.
Polypharmacy increases the risk of noncompliance and nonadherence.

19. (A) Drug adherence intervention strategy.
To ensure improved adherence to medication, the acronym SIMPLE is used when conducting interventions to improve drug adherence. SIMPLE stands for Simplifying the drug regimen, Imparting knowledge of the importance of drug adherence, Modifying patient beliefs and human behavior, Providing communication and trust, Leaving the bias and Evaluating drug adherence.

20. (A) Use of PHQ-9.
The PHQ-9 is a self-assessment tool that screens for depression, not adherence to drug regimens. Evaluation of adherence to drug regime involves using adherence scales, such as Morisky-4, asking about adherence behavior in every visit, reviewing medication containers and refill dates, and self-reporting.

21. (B) Rhabdomyolysis.
Baycol is a brand name for cerivastatin, an HMG-CoA reductase inhibitor. It was manufactured by Bayer A.G. and recalled in 2001, four years after its release. Its adverse effects included rhabdomyolysis and AKI.

22. (D) All of the above.
Barriers to medication adherence can be classified as patient-related, socioeconomic, condition-related, health system–related and therapy-related factors. Barriers, such as misconstrued perception of disease, poor insurance coverage and frequently changing patient treatment, all contribute to lack of adherence.

23. (D) Side effects of the medication.

Drug adherence is the patient's ability to take medication for the use it was intended. Unpleasant medication side effects are therapy-related factors and not health system–related factors.

24. (A) Medications with similar names and packaging should be stored in the same location.
This is false. Medications with similar names and packaging should be stored in relatively different areas. Inventory should be limited to prevent overcrowding, adequate lighting should always be maintained, and medication should be kept at eye level with labels facing outward. Separating inventory is of great importance, as it reduces the occurrence of medication errors.

25. (A) Wrong-dose error.
The prescription contains a trailing zero, and this can lead to a tenfold increase in the strength of drug dosage and cause harmful consequences. Trailing zeros and leading decimal points should be avoided to prevent wrong-dose errors. The use of error-prone abbreviations should also be avoided to prevent medication errors.

26. (C) Call the primary care physician for clarification.
When a technician is unable to decipher a prescription, the primary care physician or prescriber should be contacted for further clarification. It is inappropriate to reject the prescription, give OTC medication advice or interpret the prescription arbitrarily.

27. (B) It is also known as a blended unit dose.
A modified unit dose is a kind of unit-dose system in which a patient is given up to a month's supply of medication, as opposed to a single dose. It is also known as a bingo or blister card and is different from a blended unit dose in which medications to be taken at the same time are packaged together.

28. (C) PRN order – Given at the same time daily, based on physician's direction.

This pair is incorrectly matched. A PRN order is given only as needed or in response to a defined medical condition or parameter. A scheduled order is given at the same time each day, based on directions from the patient's physician.

29. (D) Rubber.
Urethral catheters are not made from rubber. They're made from silicone, polyurethane or latex and are inserted through the ureter into the bladder in a process known as catheterization. This process allows urine to drain from the bladder for collection and may be used to inject liquids into the bladder for the diagnosis and treatment of some conditions. Catheters come in different sizes, ranging from 8 Fr to 36 Fr.

30. (B) 18G – Pink.
This pair is incorrectly matched. A 14G cannula usually comes in orange, 16G is gray and 18G is green. These are wide-bore cannulas, useful in trauma cases or when quick fluid transfusion is required. 20G and 22G cannulas are pink and blue respectively and are used for normal IV access in older children and adults. 24G and 26G cannulas are used for neonates, children and the elderly. They are yellow and violet, respectively.

31. (A) It is unique for every new drug produced.
This is true. The NDC is a unit and permanent code assigned by the FDA for every new drug that enters the market. According to federal law, each prescription medicine must have this code, which is the letters NDC followed by three unique sets of numbers. For example, the NDC number for Norvasc (amlodipine) is NDC 0069-1520-68. It is different from the national formulary, a database of officially recognized drug names.

32. (D) Color of the medication.
Medication color is not part of the National Drug Code. The NDC is a unique and permanent code assigned to each new drug that enters the marketplace. It identifies the drug formulation, the manufacturer and distributor of the drug and the size and type of its packaging.

33. (C) NDC 03261-559-28.
The NDC of each prescription medicine is written as NDC followed by three sets of specific numbers. For example, the NDC number for Plavix (clopidogrel) is NDC 63653-1171-6.

34. (B) The NDC number is usually a 10-digit code.
This is correct. The NDC for every over-the-counter prescription medication is a 10-digit number. A drug is removed from the NDC directory when it is removed from the market. Drug companies inform the FDA if they no longer plan to produce or sell a drug, and it is removed from the NDC directory once the drug reaches its end marketing date.

35. (D) 1 g = 1,000 mcg.
This measuring conversion is false.
1 g = 1,000 mg
1 mg = 1,000 mcg
1 mg = 0.001 g
1 kg = 1,000 g

36. (A) The NDC directory is updated daily.
This is true. The NDC directory is updated by the FDA daily as new products are compounded. Not all products listed in the NDC directory are drugs as defined by federal law, and not every drug is listed in the NDC directory. For instance, animal drugs and blood products are not listed in the NDC directory.

37. (B) Recall of a drug or violative product that can cause reversible health consequences.
A Class II drug recall involves the recall of drugs whose use or exposure can cause reversible adverse health effects. Mislabeling of products, provision of incorrect safety information, and precaution and contamination of sterile nonophthalmic products are all examples of a Class II drug recall.

38. (C) Organ toxicity at high dose.
This is not a criterion used to identify hazardous drugs. Drugs are identified as hazardous or potentially hazardous based on the following six criteria:

– Teratogenicity, the ability to cause fetal malformations
– Carcinogenicity, the ability to cause cancer in humans, animal models or both
– Genotoxicity, the ability to cause an alteration in genetic material
– Potential to cause fertility impairment
– Toxic to organs at low doses
– New drugs that mimic existing hazardous drugs in structure or toxicity

39. (D) Powdered gloves.
Powdered gloves are not part of personal protective equipment (PPE). Individuals are advised to use PPE when handling or receiving hazardous materials. Typically, PPE consists of boots, a respirator (usually a HEPA mask), hair covers, face shields, coated gowns and powder-free, impermeable gloves.

40. (D) None of the above.
None of these statements is false. Shoe covers, head covers and hair covers (including covers for beard and mustache, if applicable) should be worn in areas where hazardous drugs are being compounded. Apart from protecting workers from contact with residues from these materials, they also prevent contamination of the drug being compounded by microbes and particulate matter. They should not be worn outside the compounding area to prevent exposing unprotected workers to these substances.

41. (A) Respirators protect against gases and vapors.
This is untrue. A NIOSH-certified N95 mask or higher is sufficient to protect against airborne particles when respiratory protection is required. However, these respirators offer no protection against vapors and gases and provide little protection against direct liquid splashes.

42. (C) Gloves with long cuffs should be placed under the cuff of the gown.
Two pairs of American Society for Testing and Materials (ASTM)-tested chemotherapy gloves should be worn when administering, compounding, managing spills and disposing of hazardous drugs. For sterile preparations, the outer gloves should be sterile. Inner gloves should be worn under the

gown cuff, while outer gloves or gloves with long cuffs should be worn over the gown cuff.

43. (C) Surgical scrubs and cloth laboratory coats are ideal outerwear when handling hazardous drugs.
This is false. Surgical scrubs, cloth laboratory coats or other absorbent materials are not appropriate outerwear when handling hazardous drugs because they allow the permeation of hazardous drugs. They can also hold spilled drugs against the skin, thereby increasing exposure.

44. (D) None of the above.
Many hazardous drugs can irritate eyes, skin and mucous membranes, so it is necessary to wear appropriate eye and face protection when handling these materials. Depending on the setting, face shields, goggles or full facepiece respirators may be used alone or in combination to protect the face and eyes.

45. (A) First aid box.
A first aid box is not a component of a spill kit used during exposure to hazardous drugs. Facilities that deal with hazardous substances are required to have spill kits, which may come in handy during the cleanup and containment of hazardous materials. Contents of a spill kit include waste containers, PPE, warning signs to ward off traffic from the area of the spill, disposable brushes and scoops, absorbent gauze and pads, powders for solidifying liquids, and a deactivating agent like sodium hypochlorite.

46. (C) Filing an incident report is relevant only for large-scale exposures.
This is true. Workers may be exposed to hazardous materials at any point during their handling. Hence it is important to know the potential hazards associated with these products. This information can be found in the Materials Safety Data Sheet, including information about safe handling procedures, proper cleanup and first aid. An individual exposed may be required to file an incident report no matter the size of the exposure.

47. (A) MMDLXXI.
MM = 2,000

D = 500
L = 50
XX = 20
I = 1

48. (B) 56.
The formula for calculating dose is:
D/H × V

D = 500 mg
H = 250 mg
V = 2
500 mg/250 mg × 2 = 4 tablets daily
4 tablets × 14 days = 56 tablets

49. (B) 42.
Formula is D/H × V
D = 0.5 g = 500 mg
H = 250 mg
V = 3

500 mg/250 mg × 3 times = 6 capsules daily
6 tablets × 7 days = 42 capsules

50. (B) 10.
Formula is H/V = D/X

H = 250 mg
V = 5 mL
D = 500 mg
X = unknown

250 mg/5 mL = 500 mg/X
250 mg X = 2,500 mgmL
X = 2,500 mgmL/250 mg

X = 10 mL

51. (C) 0.25.
Formula is H/V = D/X
H = 40,000 units
V = 1 mL
D = 10,000 units
X = unknown

40,000 units/1mL = 10,000 units/X
X40, 000 units = 10,000 units mL
X = 10,000 units mL/40,000 units
X = ¼ mL
X = 0.25 mL

52. (B) 7.5.
Formula is H/V = D/X

H = 10,000 units
V = 1.5 mL
D = 50,000 units
X = unknown

10,000 units/1.5 mL = 50,000 units/X
X10,000 units = 75,000 units mL
X = 75,000 units mL/10,000 units
X = 7.5 mL

53. (B) 16.

Formula is D/H × V.

H = 80 mg
V = 2 mL
D = 60 mg

X = unknown
60 mg/80 mg × 2 mL

3/4 × 2 mL = 1.5 mL per dose

1.5 mL per dose × 3 times daily = 4.5 mL
4.5 mL × 7 days = 31.5 mL approximately 32 mL

If 2 mL = 1 ampoule
32 mL = 16 ampoules

54. (B) 0.5.
Formula is $H/V = D/X$.

H = 0.4 mg
V = 1 mL
D = 0.2 mg
X = unknown

0.4 mg/1 mL = 0.2 mg/X
X = 0.2 mgmL/0.4 mg
X = 0.5 mL.

55. (C) 0.75.
Formula is $H/V = D/X$.

H = 10,000 units
V = 1 mL
D = 7,500 units
X = unknown

10,000 units/1 mL = 7,500 units/X
X10, 000 units = 7,500 units mL
X = 7,500 units mL/10,000 units
X = 0.75 mL

56. (A) Phenelzine.
This patient is experiencing a hypertensive crisis caused by a potentiation of his MAOI and tyramine found in fermented foods like cured meats and aged cheeses.

57. (B) Levodopa and carbidopa.
In synergy, two drugs work together to bring about an effect that is greater than if the drugs were given individually. Levodopa is often prescribed with carbidopa because it increases the bioavailability of levodopa in the brain by inhibiting the actions of dopa decarboxylase in peripheral tissues.

58. (B) Hyperprolactinemia.
Hyperprolactinemia is a side effect of antipsychotics that block dopamine receptors. Side effects of levodopa include dyskinesia; gastrointestinal effects like nausea and vomiting; cardiovascular effects like postural hypotension, asystole and tachycardia; and behavioral changes like agitation, hallucinations, delusion and psychosis.

59. (B) Pramipexole.
Pramipexole is a dopamine receptor agonist. Option A is a dopamine receptor blocker. Option C is exogenous dopamine, and Option D is a muscarinic receptor blocker.

60. (D) Clozapine.
This is not a first-generation antipsychotic. First-generation antipsychotics include chlorpromazine, haloperidol, fluphenazine, trifluoperazine and thioridazine. Second-generation antipsychotics, also known as atypical antipsychotics, include clozapine, quetiapine, olanzapine, ziprasidone and risperidone.

61. (A) They have a high affinity for D2 receptors.
This statement is false because, unlike first-generation antipsychotics, second-generation antipsychotics do not have a high affinity for D2 receptors. This property reduces the risk of extrapyramidal effects. Second-generation

antipsychotics also block receptors, like the alpha-adrenergic receptors, 5-HT2 receptors, H1 and D4 receptors.

62. (C) Sedation.
Sedation is common with second-generation antipsychotics that block histamine receptors (phenothiazines).

63. (B) Alpha-adrenergic receptor blockade.
Blockade of alpha-adrenergic receptors causes postural hypotension and delayed ejaculation.

64. (D) Postural hypotension.
Postural hypotension is an effect of alpha-adrenergic receptor blockade, commonly seen in second-generation (not first-generation) antipsychotics.

65. (D) TCA.
TCAs (tricyclic antidepressants) inhibit the reuptake of norepinephrine and serotonin in the brain. Examples are imipramine, amitriptyline and clomipramine.

66. (A) Filling in the prescription.
The first step toward preventing medication errors in the dispensing process is by filling in the prescription. During this process, it is important to confirm the patient's details and the prescription. In cases where the technician is unsure of the interpretation of the prescription, the physician can be called for further clarification.

67. (B) Medication reconciliation.
Medication reconciliation involves checking a prescribed medication to ensure it matches the current list of drugs a patient is taking. This process can be required during admission, transfer of care or discharge. It aims to limit the incidence of occurrence of medication errors and improve total patient well-being.

68. (C) To avoid medication errors.

Medication reconciliation used by health facilities is done to prevent medication errors. Medication reconciliation helps identify errors, such as accidental multiple listing of drugs; wrong dose, route of administration or dosing frequency of a medication; drug allergies; and medication that is inappropriate for a patient's condition.

69. (D) Drug half-life.
Pharmacokinetics refers to the study of the action of drugs within the body. It is focused on drug absorption, drug distribution, drug excretion and drug metabolism. Drug half-life is a pharmacodynamics property of a drug. It is the time taken for the plasma concentration of a drug to be reduced by 50%. Drug absorption is the amount of a drug that reaches systemic circulation. Drug excretion is the irreversible removal of a drug via bodily fluids.

70. (B) Adverse effects.
Adverse effects are serious, severe and undesired symptoms that develop after the administration of a drug. Some adverse effects may be life-threatening and require hospitalization. Forms of adverse effects include insomnia, nephrotoxicity, hepatotoxicity, bleeding diastasis and hyperactivity.

71. (A) Idiosyncratic reaction.
An idiosyncratic reaction is a unique, strange and unpredicted reaction to a drug. This type of drug reaction is not common and varies among individuals. Some idiosyncratic reactions may be life-threatening and require hospitalization. Adverse reactions are undesired effects of a drug that can cause harm to the patient.

72. (D) Niacinamide.
Penicillin, sulfa-containing drugs like sulfamethoxazole, and aspirin are notorious for hypersensitivity reactions. Hypersensitivity reactions can occur in the form of hives, rashes, itching, wheezing, swelling and wheals on the skin.

73. (D) All of the above.

An anaphylactic drug reaction is a severe form of allergic drug reaction that is life-threatening. It is a medical emergency and can cause shortness of breath, reduced cardiac output, difficulty breathing, swelling of the oropharynx and respiratory paralysis.

74. (A) Drug interaction.
Drug interaction is the interference of a drug by the effect of another drug, nutrient or laboratory test. Drug interaction is common in patients on multidrug regimens. It can occur at any point in the pharmacokinetic process of a drug, such as drug liberation, absorption, distribution, biotransformation and excretion.

75. (B) Synergism.
Synergism is the cooperative effect of two or more drugs given together that produces a stronger effect than either of the drugs when given alone. Potentiation occurs when a drug prolongs the effect of another drug. Antagonism occurs when two drugs decrease the effect of each other. An additive effect is when the combined effect of more than one agent is equal to the sum of the effects of the drugs put together.

76. (C) Trazodone.
Serotonin 5-HT2 antagonists block 5-HT2 receptors. Examples are trazodone and nefazodone.

77. (D) Ibuprofen.
An interaction with ibuprofen increases the risk of gastrointestinal bleeding and not serotonin syndrome, a form of hypertensive crisis. Serotonin syndrome occurs when an SSRI is taken with an MAOI, muscle relaxants, TCAs, St John's wort, MDMA, meperidine or dextromethorphan.

78. (B) Neostigmine.
Neostigmine is an indirect-acting cholinergic. It binds to acetylcholinesterase and prevents the degradation of acetylcholine.

79. (C) They can be used to treat myasthenia gravis.

This statement is false because organophosphates like malathion and parathion are used primarily as pesticides because of their toxicity.

80. (D) Carbachol.
Carbachol and acetylcholine stimulate both the muscarinic and nicotinic receptors. Varenicline and nicotine stimulate nicotinic receptors, while pilocarpine and bethanechol stimulate muscarinic receptors.

81. (A) Mydriasis.
Parasympathetic stimulation of the muscles in the iris causes miosis (contraction of the pupillary sphincter) and not mydriasis.

82. (D) Diaphoresis.
This is not a sign of atropine toxicity because patients with atropine toxicity are unable to sweat (anhidrosis). Anhidrosis triggers hyperthermia. Other features of atropine toxicity include hyperpyrexia, dryness of the mouth and eyes, tachycardia, constipation, acute urinary retention, blurry vision, amnesia, sedation, hallucinations, delirium, flushing and heart block.

83. (B) Urinary urgency.
Scopolamine is an anticholinergic that works on muscarinic receptors. Blockade of these receptors will cause a cessation of parasympathetic activity, like urination, peristalsis, sweating and salivation. Charlie is likely to experience urinary retention and not urgency.

84. (D) Norepinephrine.
Nonselective adrenergic agonists include norepinephrine, alpha-receptor agonist include phenylephrine, alpha 2 receptor agonists include clonidine, nonselective beta-agonists include isoproterenol, beta 1 adrenergic agonists include dobutamine, and beta 2 adrenergic agonists include albuterol.

85. (B) Miosis.
Stimulation of alpha-adrenergic receptors causes miosis and contraction of smooth muscles in blood vessels, the bladder and the prostate. Stimulation of beta-adrenergic receptors causes tachycardia and bronchoconstriction.

86. (D) Epinephrine.
Epinephrine not only stimulates both alpha and beta-adrenergic receptors in the blood vessels and heart, but it also blocks the action of anaphylaxis mediators like histamine and leukotriene.

87. (A) Albuterol.
Short-acting beta 2 agonists, like terbutaline, metaproterenol and albuterol, are unsuitable for asthma prophylaxis. They are, however, suitable for managing an acute asthma attack. Long-acting beta 2 agonists, like formoterol, olodaterol and salmeterol, are suitable for prophylaxis.

88. (C) Phenylephrine.
Phenylephrine is an alpha-adrenergic agonist that causes relaxation of the pupillary sphincter without causing cycloplegia. Anticholinergics, on the other hand, cause mydriasis and cycloplegia.

89. (A) Salbutamol.
Beta 2 adrenergic agonists like salbutamol and terbutaline cause relaxation of the smooth muscle cells in the uterus. They are useful tocolytics in obstetrics.

90. (B) Tachycardia.
This patient should be counseled on the risk of experiencing palpitations and tachycardia. These effects are caused by the action of this drug on the beta receptors in the heart.

Test 5: Questions

1. Ernie is a 67-year-old male on prazosin for benign prostatic hyperplasia. He is likely to experience which of the following side effects?

   A. Tremors
   B. Dyspnea
   C. Miosis
   D. Postural hypotension

2. Which of the following drugs is used to treat a patient with dwarfism?

   A. Mecasermin
   B. Octreotide
   C. Leuprolide
   D. Gonadorelin

3. Steven is a 27-year-old male on octreotide. He is most likely being treated for which of the following conditions?

   A. Addison's disease
   B. Acromegaly
   C. SIADH
   D. Diabetes insipidus

4. Natasha is a 35-year-old female on bromocriptine for hyperprolactinemia. She is likely to experience all except which of the following side effects?

   A. Postural hypotension
   B. Low libido
   C. Constipation
   D. Hallucinations

5. All except which of the following are uterotonics?

   A. Oxytocin
   B. Misoprostol
   C. Magnesium sulfate
   D. Ergometrine

6. All except which of the following are side effects of thioamides?

A. Agranulocytosis
B. Metallic taste
C. Vasculitis
D. Hepatitis

7. Estrogen therapy increases the risk for all except which of the following in a patient?

A. Cholelithiasis
B. Deep vein thrombosis
C. Endometrial cancer
D. Cervical cancer

8. Judy is a 29-year-old female on tamoxifen. Which of the following describes the mechanism of action of this drug?

A. GnRH agonist
B. Aromatase inhibitor
C. Estrogen receptor antagonist
D. 5α-reductase inhibitor

9. All except which of the following are symptoms of androgen toxicity?

A. Liver cancer
B. Gynecomastia
C. Infertility
D. Hypertension

10. Which of the following antiasthmatic drugs is suitable for treating acute asthma?

A. Salbutamol
B. Prednisolone
C. Zafirlukast
D. Theophylline

11. Which of the following drug pairs will produce an undesirable synergistic effect?

A. Meperidine and promethazine
B. Warfarin sodium and aspirin
C. Acetaminophen and codeine
D. Tetracycline and antacids

12. All except which of the following drug pairs will potentiate the effect of each other?

A. Penicillin and probenecid
B. Acetaminophen and codeine
C. Cimetidine and theophylline
D. Tetracycline and antacids

13. Which of the following is not a risk factor associated with drug interaction?

A. Drug abuse
B. Multiple prescribers
C. Patient compliance
D. Polypharmacy

14. The time taken for the plasma concentration of an administered drug to reduce by 50% is called ____________.

A. Half-time
B. Half-life
C. Bioavailability
D. Therapeutic index

15. Which of the following enzymes plays a major role in the biotransformation and metabolism of certain drugs?

A. Cytochrome P-450
B. Cytochrome A14
C. Cytochrome A6
D. Cytochrome B4

16. All except which of the following are patient variables that play a role in drug interaction?

A. Age
B. Sex
C. Diet
D. Genetic factors

17. Which of the following best explains the prevalence of drug-related problems commonly encountered in newborns?

A. Poorly developed enzyme system
B. Poorly developed bone marrow
C. Immature liver
D. Immature heart

18. Concerning the effect of genetic factors in drug interaction, which of the following is true?

A. They may be responsible for the development of unexpected drug responses in a patient.
B. They are associated with sexually transmitted diseases.
C. They are responsible for the development of eating disorders.
D. They are linked to obesity.

19. All except which of the following drugs should not be given concurrently with grapefruit?

A. Midazolam
B. Estrogen
C. Cyclosporine
D. Acetaminophen

20. A 20-year-old male was prescribed phenelzine to treat depression. Which foods should he avoid?

A. Rice
B. Wheat
C. Yogurt
D. Soy

21. In regards to returning medications after they have been delivered by the wholesaler, which of the following is correct?

A. No refunds are given when retailers return stocks of medications ordered.
B. Wrongly filled orders cannot be undone once received.
C. Wholesalers have policies guiding medication returns.
D. Excessive medications ordered from wholesalers cannot be returned.

22. Which of the following is correct about outdated medications?

A. Each pharmacy has a local policy for processing outdated drugs.
B. These drugs should be pulled off the shelves at regular intervals.
C. Medications dispensed to patients should be at least three months from expiration dates.
D. None of the above.

23. Concerning outdated medications, which of the following is false?

A. Wholesalers accept expired drugs for credit if they are returned within a fixed time frame.
B. Medications that cannot be returned to the wholesaler must be destroyed.
C. The CPhT ensures soon-to-expire medications are pulled off the shelves regularly.
D. A list of expired products must be compiled and sent to the wholesaler for approval.

24. Which of the following statements is false concerning the use of reverse distributors?

A. The reverse distribution comes at no cost.
B. Reverse distributors retrieve unusable medications from pharmacies and ship them to manufacturers.
C. Paperwork required by manufacturers is filled by reverse distributors.
D. Reverse distributors can track the progress of medication return to the manufacturers.

25. Which of the following classes of medicines qualifies for an overstock return?

A. Medications that are slowly moving off the shelf
B. Medications that are expired
C. Medications that are damaged
D. Bottles of medications that are opened

26. Concerning damaged products, which of the following is false?

A. Products that are damaged on delivery from the manufacturer can be returned.
B. An approval code is necessary before a manufacturer receives a damaged product.
C. Manufacturers may provide refunds to pharmacies for damaged products.
D. A patient cannot return a damaged product after its attempted use.

27. Which of the following is not a reason for medication recall?

A. Incorrect labeling
B. Market competition from other brands
C. Contamination of a batch of medications
D. Errors with the packaging of products

28. Concerning unclaimed prescriptions, which of the following is false?

A. Medications that have not been picked up by patients are to be discarded after a time frame.
B. Medications are restocked 7 to 14 days after they have been initially filled.
C. Insurance companies may need to be contacted about unclaimed prescriptions.
D. Calling patients days ahead of returning their prescription to the shelf helps reduce the number of unclaimed prescriptions.

29. You receive an order for 10 mg of epinephrine, but the inventory has a 1:1,000 solution available. What volume of drugs should be dispensed?

A. 10 mL
B. 100 mL
C. 1 mL
D. 0.001 mL

30. Which of the following pieces of information is not required for documentation when a stock of products is being returned to the wholesaler?

A. The order number of the original purchase
B. The list of other items not being returned
C. The item number of the item being returned
D. The reason the item is being returned

31. Which of the following wastes should be discarded in a yellow container?

A. Contaminated personal protective equipment
B. Fully used syringes, vials and tubings
C. Bags of hazardous drugs waste
D. All of the above

32. Which of the following items must be disposed of in a black container?

A. Resource Conservation and Recovery Act–listed wastes
B. Used personal protective equipment
C. Trace-contaminated items
D. None of the above

33. Regarding the Comprehensive Drug Abuse Prevention and Control Act, which of the following statements is untrue?

A. It is the first document ever created to address and regulate illicit substance use.
B. It provided the legal framework for the creation of the Drug Enforcement Administration.
C. Various updates have been made to the act since its inception.
D. This act provides for the acquisition, distribution and classification of controlled substances.

34. Which of the following statements is untrue about controlled substances?

A. Controlled substances are drugs with restrictions as a result of their potential to
be abused.

B. There are six schedules of controlled substances.

C. Schedules are classified based on their medicinal benefit versus their potential for abuse.

D. The Controlled Substance Act provides the Drug Enforcement Administration with the authority to classify controlled drugs into schedules.

35. Characteristics of Schedule I drugs include all except which of the following?

A. Unaccepted medical use

B. The highest potential for abuse

C. Sufficient medicinal use to justify availability as a prescription

D. Not available for prescription

36. Schedule III drugs include all except which of the following?

A. Naloxone

B. Morphine

C. Testosterone

D. Buprenorphine

37. Which of the following drugs is an example of a Schedule V drug?

A. Lomotil

B. Phenobarbital

C. Tcstosterone

D. Amphetamine

38. Which of the following is untrue about purchasing Schedule II medication?

A. Schedule II medications need to be checked in against a DEA form when they arrive at the pharmacy.
B. A pharmacy must register with the DEA to purchase a Schedule II medication
C. Schedule II drugs may be purchased through a controlled substances ordering system.
D. Schedule II drugs may be ordered by a pharmacy or other appropriate dispensary.

39. Which of the following is false concerning the purchase of scheduled substances?

A. The DEA Form 222 is a triplicate form.
B. The pharmacy retains the third sheet and sends the first and second pages to the DEA.
C. Schedule II medications should be checked in against a DEA form when they arrive in the pharmacy.
D. None of the above.

40. Which of the following is false about prescriptions?

A. Prescribers are required to include their DEA number on the prescription.
B. Schedule II prescriptions may be written for up to 90 days.
C. Schedule III prescriptions may be written for up to one year.
D. Prescribers should not exceed a 90-day supply of Schedule II drugs without assessing the patient.

41. A prescription order is as follows: Penicillin G 100,000 units/mL. The available dose is 1,000,000 units per vial. How many mL of diluent will be added to this drug?

A. 1
B. 10
C. 100
D. 0.1

42. A prescription order is as follows: Insulin lispro 14 units tid. The available dose is insulin 100 U/mL in 3 mL vials. A vial will last how long for this patient?

A. 6 days
B. 14 days
C. 7 days
D. 8 days

43. A prescription order is as follows: 1% epinephrine. How is this expressed in mg/mL?

A. 1
B. 10
C. 100
D. 0.1

44. A drug solution is presented as 20 mg/mL. What percentage of drugs is in this solution?

A. 2%
B. 0.2%
C. 20%
D. 200%

45. A prescription order comes in as 1 g in 50 mL. What is the percentage of the solution?

A. 5%
B. 50%
C. 2%
D. 20%

46. How many mg are in 5 mL of 2% solution?

A. 10
B. 100
C. 1
D. 0.1 mg

47. The physician's order is as follows: Chloramphenicol 1% ophthalmic solution, 0.2 mL in each eye for 5 days. How many milligrams will be added to each eye?

A. 1
B. 0.1
C. 2
D. 0.2

48. You are to compound 50 mL of 1:1,000 solution of furosemide with 20 mg tablets of furosemide. How many of these tablets will you need?

A. 2
B. 2.5
C. 3
D. 3.5

49. You are to compound 30 mL of a 2% solution of diazepam. How many milligrams of this drug are required?

A. 60
B. 6
C. 0.6
D. 600

50. Mark, a 15-year-old male, is on IV theophylline for severe asthma. Which of the following describes the mechanism of action of this drug?

A. Muscarinic receptor blocker
B. Beta 2 agonist
C. Mast cell stabilizer
D. Phosphodiesterase inhibitor

51. All except which of the following are inhalational corticosteroids?

A. Fluticasone
B. Flunisolide
C. Hydrocortisone
D. Budesonide

52. Which of the following is a bulk laxative?

A. Glycerol
B. Psyllium
C. Sorbitol
D. Docusate

53. John is taking senna. He is likely to experience all except which of the following side effects?

A. Abdominal cramps
B. Diarrhea
C. Dehydration
D. Tarry stools

54. All except which of the following laxatives are unsuitable for a patient with fecal impaction?

A. Bisacodyl
B. Methylcellulose
C. Glycerin
D. Sorbitol

55. Jack is on Tegretol, docusate, Tagamet and Advil. Which of the following drug-drug interactions is most likely?

   A. Tegretol-Docusate
   B. Docusate-Tagamet
   C. Tegretol-Advil
   D. Tegretol-Tagamet

56. Which of the following antibacterials is not effective in its oral form?

   A. Penicillin G
   B. Penicillin V
   C. Amoxicillin
   D. Ampicillin

57. All except which of the following drugs are susceptible to penicillinase?

   A. Amoxicillin
   B. Ticarcillin
   C. Oxacillin
   D. Piperacillin

58. Penicillin extended-release is given only via the IM route. Which of the following justifies the route of this drug's administration?

   A. It is a vesicant.
   B. It is an emulsion.
   C. It is high in dextrose.
   D. It has a small volume.

59. Which of the following statements is false about penicillins?

   A. They are bacteriostatic.
   B. They are beta-lactam antibiotics.
   C. They inhibit the synthesis of cell walls.
   D. Clavulanic acid is added to inhibit the action of penicillinase.

60. Concerning alcohol consumption and drug interaction, which of the following is correct?

A. It is an excessive depressant response when taken with sedatives.
B. Acute use by individuals who are not alcoholics may inhibit hepatic enzymes.
C. Chronic alcohol use can induce the metabolism of warfarin.
D. All of the above.

61. Smoking increases the metabolism of all except which of the following drugs?

A. Theophylline
B. Metformin
C. Diazepam
D. Amitriptyline

62. All except which of the following factors reduce the risk of drug interaction?

A. Identifying the patient's risk factors
B. Obtaining a thorough drug history
C. Administering a multidrug regimen
D. Considering therapeutic alternatives

63. Safe work practices that are put into place for the care and treatment of all patients irrespective of their known or presumed infection status are called ____________.

A. Standard precautions
B. Work safety
C. Ergonomics
D. First aid

64. Which of the following is not a standard precaution that should be observed in a pharmacy?

A. Handwashing
B. Use of personal protective equipment
C. Correct handling and disposal of waste material
D. None of the above

65. Which of the following is true concerning personal protective equipment?

A. PPE creates a physical barrier between the health worker and potentially infectious material.
B. It consists of protective gloves, gown, mask and footwear.
C. It may be disposable.
D. All of the above.

66. Technicians should clean the countertops and equipment with ____________ before they begin compounding any medication.

A. Alcohol
B. Warm water
C. Soapy water
D. Turpentine

67. Which of the following is true about handwashing?

A. Hands should be washed and sanitized before compounding medication.
B. Hands should be washed before entering the IV preparation room.
C. Hands should be washed before working in a laminar airflow hood.
D. All of the above.

68. Jane, a CPhT, is preparing an IV medication. The most important aspect of the safety precautions while preparing a sterile product is ______________.

A. Handwashing
B. Aseptic technique
C. Using 95% isopropyl alcohol to wipe down a laminar hood
D. Cleaning countertops with warm soapy water

69. Which of the following products can be retrieved for credit by reverse distribution companies?

A. Reconstituted drugs
B. Unusable Schedule II, III, IV and V controlled substances
C. Partially used bottles of medication
D. None of the above

70. Which of the following classes of medication recalls is correctly paired?

A. Class I – Medications are recalled because they may cause serious harm to a patient's health, including the risk of death.
B. Class II – Medications are recalled for reasons that are unlikely to have adverse health consequences.
C. Class III – Medications are recalled because they can cause temporary or reversible health effects.
D. None of the above

71. Which of the following household measures is not correctly paired with its corresponding laboratory measure?

A. 15 mL – 1 tablespoon
B. 2 mL – 1 teaspoon
C. 240 mL – 1 cup
D. 30 mL – 2 tablespoons

72. Which of the following terms describes the relationship between two equal ratios?

A. Proportion
B. Rate
C. Decimal
D. Fraction

73. Which of the following prescription abbreviations is incorrectly matched?

A. a.m. – Morning
B. Stat – Immediately
C. BID – Once daily
D. QID – Four times daily

74. Which of the following dosage forms is correctly matched?
   A. APP – Ointment
   B. C – Suppository
   C. UNG – Capsule
   D. TAB – Tablet

75. All except which of the following cephalosporins have extensive coverage against gram-negative infections?
   A. Cefuroxime
   B. Cefazolin
   C. Ceftriaxone
   D. Cefepime

76. Which of the following antibiotics is not a cell wall inhibitor?
   A. Vancomycin
   B. Fosfomycin
   C. Azithromycin
   D. Daptomycin

77. Which of the following antibiotics is associated with a risk of cyanosis and heart failure in infants?
   A. Imipenem
   B. Clindamycin
   C. Chloramphenicol
   D. Tetracycline

78. All except which of the following antibiotics are unsuitable for use in children?
   A. Tetracycline
   B. Chloramphenicol
   C. Levofloxacin
   D. Gentamicin

79. Significant side effects of aminoglycosides include all except ___________.

A. Ototoxicity
B. Nephrotoxicity
C. Cardiotoxicity
D. Allergic skin reactions

80. All except which of the following drugs increase the risk of renal failure?

A. Sulfamethoxazole
B. Amikacin
C. Erythromycin
D. Tetracycline

81. You are monitoring a patient who is on an IV infusion of vancomycin. You notice that the patient appears flushed and red. Blood pressure and heart rate are, however, normal. Which of the following interventions is most appropriate?

A. Stop the infusion and give IV hydrocortisone.
B. Flush the line with normal saline.
C. Slow down the infusion.
D. Do nothing and observe.

82. A patient with a penicillin allergy will probably be allergic to all except which of the following drugs?

A. Bactrim
B. Rocephin
C. Vancocin
D. Ceclor

83. All except which of the following antibiotics increase sensitivity to the sun?

A. Doxycycline
B. Ciprofloxacin
C. Trimethoprim
D. Gentamicin

84. Which of the following anti-TB drugs causes orange discoloration of bodily fluids?

A. Isoniazid
B. Ethambutol
C. Rifampin
D. Pyrazinamide

85. Which of the following anti-TB drugs needs a co-prescription with pyridoxine?

A. Isoniazid
B. Ethambutol
C. Rifampin
D. Pyrazinamide

86. All except which of the following anti-TB drugs require serial monitoring of liver function?

A. Isoniazid
B. Ethambutol
C. Rifampin
D. Pyrazinamide

87. Which of the following anti-TB drugs requires serial ophthalmic examinations?

A. Isoniazid
B. Ethambutol
C. Rifampin
D. Pyrazinamide

88. Which of the following statements about vancomycin is correct?

A. It has a broad spectrum.
B. It is bacteriostatic.
C. It inhibits transglycosylation.
D. It can be absorbed from the gut.

89. All except which of the following are nephrotoxic drugs?

   A. Probenecid
   B. Vancomycin
   C. Erythromycin
   D. Trimethoprim

90. All except which of the following classes of antifungals block the permeability of a fungi's cell membrane?

   A. Terbinafine
   B. Echinocandins
   C. Azoles
   D. Polyenes

Test 5: Answers and Explanations

1. (D) Postural hypotension.
Prazosin is an alpha 1 adrenergic receptor blocker. Its side effects include profound postural hypotension and reflex tachycardia.

2. (A) Mecasermin.
Mecasermin is a growth hormone agonist used to treat patients with dwarfism from growth hormone deficiency.

3. (B) Acromegaly.
Octreotide is a growth hormone antagonist used to treat patients with acromegaly caused by excessive secretion of growth hormone.

4. (B) Low libido.
Bromocriptine is a partial D2 receptor agonist. It is used to treat hyperprolactinemia, a disease that is characterized by amenorrhea, galactorrhea, low libido and infertility. As a dopamine agonist, side effects include nausea and vomiting; cardiovascular effects like postural hypotension, asystole and tachycardia; and behavioral changes like agitation, hallucinations, delusions and psychosis.

5. (C) Magnesium sulfate.
Magnesium sulfate relaxes uterine muscles and is used to prevent premature labor. It is a tocolytic. Uterotonics increase the strength and frequency of uterine contractions. They are useful in obstetrics. Examples include oxytocin, misoprostol, mifepristone, ergometrine and carboprost.

6. (B) Metallic taste.
Metallic taste is not a side effect of thioamides. Thioamides inhibit the synthesis of thyroxine by blocking the action of peroxidase and blocking iodination. They also block the conversion of T4 to T3. Examples are propylthiouracil and methimazole. Side effects include agranulocytosis, rashes, vasculitis, hepatitis and hypoprothrombinemia.

7. (D) Cervical cancer.
Estrogen does not increase the risk for cervical cancer. But it does increase the risk for breast cancer, endometrial cancer, stroke, myocardial infarction, deep vein thrombosis, hypertriglyceridemia, migraine headaches, gallbladder disease and hypertension.

8. (C) Estrogen receptor antagonist.
Tamoxifen is an estrogen receptor antagonist used to treat breast cancer. An example of a GnRH agonist is danazol. An example of an aromatase inhibitor is anastrozole, and an example of a 5α-reductase inhibitor is finasteride.

9. (D) Hypertension.
Androgen toxicity in males causes feminization characterized by gynecomastia, infertility and shrinkage of the testes. High doses in both sexes increase the risk of cholestatic jaundice and liver cancer.

10. (A) Salbutamol.
Nebulized salbutamol is suitable for treating acute asthma. It is a short-acting beta 2 agonist.

11. (B) Warfarin sodium and aspirin.
The combination of warfarin sodium and aspirin causes an undesirable synergistic effect that increases the risk of bleeding diastasis, as these two drugs prevent clotting and enhance blood loss. Synergism occurs when the effect of two or more drugs when given together has a stronger effect than when either of the drugs is given alone.

12. (D) Tetracycline and antacids.
Antacids inhibit the absorption of tetracycline from the small intestine. The combination of tetracycline and antacids is an example of antagonism. Drug potentiation occurs when the effect of a drug is prolonged by another drug. Drug potentiation effect occurs in drug combinations, such as penicillin and probenecid, acetaminophen and codeine, and cimetidine and theophylline.

13. (C) Patient compliance.
Patient compliance is a patient's ability to adhere to drug therapy. It is not a risk factor associated with drug interaction. Polypharmacy occurs when patients take numerous drugs that may be from different prescribers, which is common in surgical inpatients who may take more than 10 medications at a time. Drug abuse is the use of a drug for other purposes than it was prescribed. The risk factors associated with drug interaction include drug abuse, multiple prescribers, polypharmacy, patient noncompliance, multiple pharmacological effects and nonprescription drug use.

14. (B) Half-life.
The time taken for the plasma concentration of an administered drug to reduce by 50% is known as the half-life. Bioavailability is the measurement of the rate at which a drug is absorbed and the total amount of drug that reaches the systemic circulation from the dosage form administered. The therapeutic index is the measure of the margin of safety of a drug.

15. (A) Cytochrome P-450.
The oxidative biotransformation and metabolism of certain drugs are carried out by a system of enzymes known as the cytochrome P-450. These enzymes have been linked to many drug interactions. The cytochrome P-450 enzyme system can be induced or inhibited by a variety of substances that can affect the metabolism of drugs.

16. (B) Sex.
Drug interaction is the interference of the effect of a drug by another drug, food or laboratory test. Patient variables that play a role in drug interaction include age, diet, genetic factors, disease and conditions of the patient, alcohol and smoking. These factors play a role in the response of patients to certain drugs. Sex plays no role in drug interactions.

17. (A) Poorly developed enzyme system.
Drug-related problems are commonly encountered in newborns because they have a poorly developed enzyme system and immature renal function.

18. (A) They may be responsible for the development of unexpected drug responses in a patient.
Genetic factors play a role in the development of unexpected drug responses in patients. Some patients may metabolize drugs faster, and some more slowly. This can cause a lack of therapeutic effects or an increase in unwanted side effects.

19. (D) Acetaminophen.
Grapefruit juice interacts with some drugs metabolized by the cytochrome-p450 enzymes. Cyclosporine, midazolam, estrogen, triazolam, calcium channel blockers and simvastatin should not be taken concurrently with grapefruit juice. Grapefruit juice induces the enzyme system of the cytochrome p-450 and causes rapid metabolism of these drugs, leading to reduced therapeutic effects. Drug dose adjustments may be needed in these cases.

20. (C) Yogurt.
Monoamine oxidase inhibitors are used to treat depression and anxiety in some patient groups. Patients on monoamine oxidative (MAO) inhibitors should avoid yogurt, wine, cured meat and cheese to avoid potential toxic effects. These food sources contain tyramine, which potentiates the effects of MAO inhibitors. A combination of this diet and the MAO inhibitors will cause a potentially dangerous drug-food reaction that results in a hypertensive crisis.

21. (C) Wholesalers have policies guiding medication returns.
This is correct. In some situations, goods received from wholesalers may be expired, damaged, in excess or incorrect orders. These drugs may be returned to the wholesalers for credit. However, wholesalers have policies guiding what medications may be returned, and these rules have to be followed properly to receive credit for returns.

22. (C) Medications dispensed to patients should be at least three months from expiration dates.

This is correct. Because medications are usually issued to patients in 90-day supplies, the expiration date of a medication must be at least three months away for these patients. CPhTs should pull medications from the shelf two to three months before their date of expiration.

23. (B) Medications that cannot be returned to the wholesaler must be destroyed.
Generally, wholesalers accept outdated drugs for credit when they are returned within a specific time limit, usually two to three months before and after the manufacturer's expiration date. Medications that cannot be returned to the wholesaler may be sent to a reverse distributor for credit.

24. (A) Reverse distribution comes at no cost.
This is false. The use of the services of reverse distributors comes at a cost, which is usually a percentage of the refund. This fee is automatically deducted from the final amount to be refunded to the pharmacy.

25. (A) Medications that are slowly moving off the shelf.
Generally, if a drug package has not been opened or damaged and will not expire for at least another 12 months, the pharmacy may send the drug back to the wholesaler. Drugs that are moving slowly off the shelves or have been ordered in excess can be returned.

26. (D) A patient cannot return a damaged product after its attempted use.
If patients receive a product and discover that it is damaged after attempting to use it, they may return it to the pharmacy for a replacement. The pharmacy can contact the manufacturer for a replacement or credit after replacing the medication from available stock.

27. (B) Market competition from other brands.
Market competition is not a reason for a medication recall. The FDA requires manufacturers to recall products with incorrect labeling, package or production errors, contamination of a particular batch of medications or any other error that breaches the FDA or manufacturer's set guidelines.

28. (A) Medications that have not been picked up by patients are to be discarded after a time frame.
This is false. Medications that have not been picked up by patients need to be returned to the shelf after a few days for use by other patients. Generally, most pharmacies have a policy that requires medications to be reshelved after 7 to 14 days.

29. (A) 10 mL.
Remember that 1:1,000 is the same as 1 mg/mL.
To calculate the amount of drug to be dispensed, divide the order by the stock 10 mg ÷ 1 mg/mL = 10 mL.

30. (B) List of other items not being returned.
A list of other items not being returned is not required. When a product to be returned is being shipped to the wholesaler, the following should be documented and shipped along with the product to the wholesaler: original purchase order number, the item number of the item being returned, the quantity to be returned and the reason for return.

31. (D) All of the above.
Properly labeled, spill-proof and leakproof containers of nonreactive plastics are required for waste disposal in areas where hazardous wastes are generated. These plastics are color coded and can be yellow or black. Fully used syringes, vials, tubing and trace-contaminated items can be disposed of in a yellow, well-labeled container. Partially used or expired hazardous substances may also be disposed of in yellow containers if they are not considered Resource Conservation and Recovery Act–regulated materials.

32. (A) Resource Conservation and Recovery Act–listed wastes.
All wastes generated from RCRA-listed materials must be placed in black RCRA-approved containers. Hazardous wastes must be properly manifested and transported by federally permitted hazardous waste transporters to a standard waste storage, treatment and disposal facility.

33. (A) It is the first document ever created to address and regulate illicit substance use.
This is untrue. The Comprehensive Drug Abuse Prevention and Control Act provides for the classification, acquisition, distribution, verification and registration of prescribers and the appropriate requirements for recordkeeping for controlled substances. This act was created to replace similar acts that previously existed, including the Harrison Narcotics Tax Act.

34. (B) There are six schedules of controlled substances.
This is untrue. There are five schedules of controlled substances, each having various prescription guidelines that are based on their medicinal benefit counterbalanced by their potential for abuse as determined by the DEA and individual state legislative branches.

35. (C) Sufficient medicinal use to justify availability as a prescription.
Characteristics of Schedule 1 drugs do not include sufficient medicinal use to justify availability as a prescription. Schedule I (CI) substances have the highest potential for abuse and are unacceptable for medical use. They are not prescription drugs. Examples of these medications include heroin, LSD and methaqualone (quaaludes).

36. (B) Morphine.
Morphine is an example of a Schedule II drug. These drugs have a high potential for abuse, with sufficient medicinal use to justify their availability as prescription. Schedule III drugs are medications with a moderate potential for misuse, abuse or dependence. Examples include suboxone (buprenorphine and naloxone), testosterone (androgel) and codeine when combined with a cough suppressant or acetaminophen in a solid dosage form (capsules, tablets, etc.).

37. (A) Lomotil.
Schedule V is made of drugs with a low potential for abuse or misuse. Examples include antidiarrheal medications that contain limited amounts of an opiate like Lomotil (atropine and diphenoxylate). Cough medicines that contain limited amounts of codeine are also classified as Schedule V drugs.

38. (D) Schedule II drugs may be ordered by a pharmacy or other appropriate dispensary.
This is untrue. Schedule II drugs have stringent requirements. A pharmacist must authorize the purchase of these drugs, and the purchase must be executed on a triplicate DEA 222 order form or through a controlled substance ordering system using an electronic 222 form.

39. (B) The pharmacy retains the third sheet and sends the first and second pages to the DEA.
This is false. The DEA Form 222 is a triplicate form. The pharmacy retains the third sheet and sends the first two pages to the wholesaler, which keeps the first page for its records while sending the second page to the DEA.

40. (C) Schedule III prescriptions may be written for up to one year.
This is false. Schedule III and IV medications may be written for up to a six-month supply, including refills on the original medication. Schedule II medications may be written for up to 90 days, without including refills. Prescribers should not exceed a 90-day supply of Schedule II drugs without reviewing the patient again.

41. (B) 10.
Formula is H/V = D/X.

H = 100,000 units
V = 1 mL
D = 1,000,000 units
X = unknown

100,000 units/1 mL = 1,000,000/X
X = 1,000,000 units mL/100,000 units
X = 10 mL

42. (C) 7 days.
Formula is H/V = D/X.

H = 100 units
V = 1 mL
D = 14 units
X = unknown

100 units/1 mL = 14 units/X
X = 14 units mL/100 units
X = 0.14 mL per dose
Three times a day = 0.14 mL × 3 = 0.42 mL per day
Since a vial is 3 mL, the duration is 3 mL/0.42 mL = 7.14 days = 7 days.

43. (B) 10.

1% = 1 g in 100 mL
Convert g to mg = 1,000 mg
1,000 mg/100 mL = 10 mg/mL

44. (A) 2%.
Since a w in v solution is expressed as g in 100 mL, convert 20 mg to g = 0.02 g.

0.02g × 100 mL/1× 100 mL = 2 g/100 mL = 2%

45. (C) 2%.
Weight in volume is expressed in grams per 100 mL.
Since the gram is in the right unit, we have to express 50 mL in 100 mL by multiplying both the numerator and denominator by 2.

1 g × 2 mL/50 mL × 2 mL = 2 gmL/100 mLmL
= 2 g/mL = 2%

46. (B) 100.
2% solution = 2 g/100 mL
Convert g to mg = 2,000 mg/100 mL = 20 mg/mL

20 mg/mL × 5 mL = 100 mg

47. (C) 2.
Remember that a 1% solution = 1 g/100 mL
Convert grams to mg = 1,000 mg/100 mL = 10 mg/mL.
The number of grams in 0.2 mL =

XmL = 10 mg × 0.2 mL
Xml = 2 mgmL
X = 2 mg

48. (B) 2.5.

Remember that 1:1,000 = 1 g/1,000 mL.

50 mL of furosemide will require:

1g/1,000mL = X/50 mL
X = 0.05 g = 50 mg

Since 1 tablet = 20 mg
50 mg = 2.5 tablets

49. (D) 600.
A 2% solution is equal to 2 g/100 mL.

2 g/100 mL = X g/30 mL

Xg = 30 mL ×2 g/100 mL
X = 0.6 g = 600 mg

50. (D) Phosphodiesterase inhibitor.
Theophylline is a methylxanthine that inhibits the action of phosphodiesterase (PDE), an enzyme that breaks down vAMP to AMP. By

blocking this enzyme, they increase concentrations of cAMP, which initiates relaxation of smooth muscle.

51. (C) Hydrocortisone.
Hydrocortisone is a short-acting corticosteroid that is given intravenously. Examples of inhalational corticosteroids include dexamethasone, fluticasone, flunisolide, budesonide and beclomethasone.

52. (B) Psyllium.
Psyllium is a bulk laxative that promotes peristalsis by bulking stools up with insoluble fiber. Other examples are polycarbophil and methylcellulose.

53. (D) Tarry stools.
Senna is a stimulant laxative that stimulates peristalsis by irritating the gut mucosa. Other examples are bisacodyl, sodium picosulfate and glycerol. Side effects include abdominal cramps, vomiting, diarrhea, nausea and tolerance. Tarry stools are not a side effect of senna.

54. (C) Glycerin.
Glycerin is a stool softener that softens stool by lubricating the rectum and anus. Other examples include docusate and mineral oil. It is suitable for patients with fecal impaction, anal fissures and hemorrhoids.

55. (D) Tegretol-Tagamet.
Tagamet is a trade name for cimetidine, an H2-receptor antagonist. This drug induces and inhibits certain cytochrome p450 enzymes. Because of this, cimetidine has interactions with more than a hundred drugs, of which anticonvulsants (such as Tegretol or carbamazepine) are likely.

56. (A) Penicillin G.
Penicillin G is not effective in its oral form because large amounts have to be taken for it to exert a therapeutic effect. It is effective in its IV and IM forms.

57. (C) Oxacillin.

Oxacillin contains a penicillinase inhibitor that blocks the action of this enzyme on the drug. It is resistant to penicillinase. Other penicillinase-resistant penicillins include cloxacillin, dicloxacillin and nafcillin.

58. (A) It is a vesicant.
Penicillins with extended-release contain either epinephrine or procaine, potent vasoconstrictors that slow down the rate of absorption of the drug into the systemic circulation and therefore control release. These drugs are vesicants that can cause phlebitis if they are given IV. They must be given through the IM route.

59. (A) They are bacteriostatic.
This statement is false because penicillins are bactericidal. This means that they kill bacteria directly without depending on the host's immune system.

60. (D) All of the above.
Chronic alcohol consumption can cause an excessive depressant response when taken with sedatives. Acute use of alcohol by individuals who are not alcoholics may inhibit hepatic enzymes. Chronic alcohol use can induce the metabolism of warfarin, phenytoin and tolbutamide because it increases the activity of liver enzymes.

61. (B) Metformin.
Cigarette smoking causes an induction of the cytochrome p-450 enzymes. This causes the rapid metabolism of certain drugs, but not Metformin. The metabolism of theophylline, diazepam, amitriptyline and chlorpromazine can be induced by cigarette smoking. These drugs are rapidly metabolized, and their therapeutic effects are decreased. These effects are more pronounced in young and middle-aged patients than in the older patient population.

62. (C) Administering a multidrug regimen.
Multidrug regimen administration and polypharmacy increase the potential for drug interactions. Factors that reduce the risk of drug interaction include identifying patient risk factors, obtaining a thorough drug history, considering therapeutic alternatives and refraining from the complex therapeutic regimen.

63. (A) Standard precautions.
Standard precautions are safe work practices put in place for the care and safety of all patients, irrespective of their known or presumed infection status. Standard precautions are the minimum level of safety precautions that are put in place in a health-care setting to limit the spread of infection.

64. (D) None of the above.
Standard universal precautions that are used for infection control include handwashing, using PPE, correct handling and disposal of waste, appropriate cleaning of patient care equipment and hygienic environmental control. These steps are necessary to limit the spread of infection within the workspace and among patients.

65. (D) All of the above.
Personal protective equipment is a safety apparatus that creates a physical barrier that protects health workers from potentially infectious material. Most PPE is disposable and includes gloves, gowns, goggles, masks and footwear. PPE is used for body substance isolation and protects health personnel from harmful and potentially dangerous materials.

66. (A) Alcohol.
The CPhT should clean the countertops and equipment with 75% isopropyl alcohol before and after compounding any medication. The countertops and equipment should be cleaned first in the morning and throughout the day to maintain a clean and safe environment. This is to prevent contamination of compounded medication. Warm water, soapy water and turpentine should not be used to clean countertops or equipment.

67. (D) All of the above.
Handwashing is a standard safety precaution. CPhTs must wash their hands before preparing and compounding medication, before and after entering the IV preparation room, and before and after working in a laminar airflow hood.

68. (B) Aseptic technique.

Aseptic technique is the most important aspect of preparing a sterile product, above all other methods. It is the most cost-effective method too.

69. (B) Unusable Schedule II, III, IV and V controlled substances.
Some products are not eligible to reverse distributors, wholesalers or manufacturers. They include reconstituted or compounded drug products and partially used bottles of medications. Unusable Schedule II, III, IV and V controlled substances are eligible for reverse distribution.

70. (A) Class I – Medications are recalled because they may cause serious harm to a patient's health, including the risk of death.
Recalls are classified into three classes:
Class I, when they may cause serious harm to a patient's health, including the risk of death; Class II, when they can cause temporary or reversible health effects; and Class III, for reasons that are unlikely to have adverse health consequences.

71. (B) 2 mL – 1 teaspoon.
This is not correctly paired. 5 mL of fluid is approximately equal to 1 teaspoon. Although household measures are not accurate enough for health-care professionals to use in the calculation of drug dosages in pharmacies and hospitals, they are still used for medications at home.

72. (A) Proportion.
A proportion shows the relationship between two equal ratios. It may be expressed as 3:6 : 1:2 or 3:6 = 1:2.
These ratios are equal because multiplying 1 and 2 by 3 will yield 3 and 6, respectively. In a proportion, the product of the two outer terms (known as the extremes) will yield the same result as multiplying the two inner terms (known as the means).

73. (C) BID – Once daily.
This is incorrectly matched. The abbreviation BID, when attached to a prescription, indicates that the medication should be administered two times each day.

74. (D) TAB – Tablet.
This is correctly matched. Dosage forms may be abbreviated when written on medications and the technician needs to know what each short form represents.

75. (B) Cefazolin.
Cefazolin is a first-generation cephalosporin with a wide coverage against gram-positive bacteria. However, it has low coverage against gram-negative bacteria compared to the other generations.

76. (C) Azithromycin.
Azithromycin is not a cell wall inhibitor. It is a macrolide. It inhibits the synthesis of proteins in bacteria. Cell wall inhibitors include penicillins, cephalosporins, carbapenems, aztreonam, vancomycin, fosfomycin, bacitracin, cycloserine and daptomycin.

77. (C) Chloramphenicol.
Chloramphenicol increases the risk of gray baby syndrome (characterized by cyanosis, anemia and heart failure) in infants.

78. (D) Gentamicin.
Gentamicin may be used in children. Tetracycline increases the risk of dysplasia and discoloration of the enamel; chloramphenicol increases the risk of gray baby syndrome; and levofloxacin, a fluoroquinolone, increases the risk of tendinitis.

79. (C) Cardiotoxicity.
Aminoglycoside is a protein synthesis inhibitor. Examples include gentamicin, kanamycin, tobramycin, neomycin and amikacin. Side effects include ototoxicity, nephrotoxicity and allergic skin reactions. Cardiotoxicity is not a side effect of aminoglycoside.

80. (C) Erythromycin.

Erythromycin is a macrolide. It does not increase the risk of nephrotoxicity, as it is not a nephrotoxic drug. Side effects of erythromycin include skin rashes, GI distress, eosinophilia, hepatitis and inhibition of CYP450 enzymes.

81. (C) Slow down the infusion.
The most appropriate intervention is to slow down the rate of infusion. This patient is experiencing red man syndrome, a side effect of vancomycin. It occurs when there is a massive release of histamines. A common cause is a rapid IV infusion of the drug.

82. (C) Vancocin.
A patient with a penicillin allergy can also be allergic to cephalosporins and sulfa-containing drugs. Bactrim is a brand name for trimethoprim/sulfamethoxazole. Rocephin is a brand name for ceftriaxone. Vancocin is a brand name for vancomycin, and Ceclor is a brand name for cefaclor, a second-generation cephalosporin.

83. (D) Gentamicin.
Gentamicin does not increase sensitivity to the sun. Drug groups that increase photosensitivity include fluoroquinolones, trimethoprim and tetracyclines.

84. (C) Rifampin.
Side effects of rifampin include orange staining of urine, sweat and tears. Other side effects include nephritis, hepatitis, rashes and thrombocytopenia. It also induces certain CYP450 enzymes and therefore quickens the elimination of a lot of drugs, including contraceptives, terbinafine, ketoconazole, anticonvulsants, methadone and warfarin.

85. (A) Isoniazid.
Side effects of isoniazid include insomnia, peripheral neuritis, restlessness and tremors. These symptoms are prevented by prescribing the drug with pyridoxine.

86. (B) Ethambutol.

Isoniazid, pyrazinamide and rifampin increase the risk of hepatitis. Because of this, serial monitoring of liver function is required.

87. (B) Ethambutol.
Ethambutol increases the risk of optic neuritis, reduced visual acuity and color blindness. Because of this, it requires serial ophthalmic examinations.

88. (C) It inhibits transglycosylation.
This is correct. Vancomycin has a narrow spectrum of action and is only used to treat infections by gram-positive bacteria resistant to methicillin and penicillin. It is a bactericidal drug that kills bacteria by inhibiting transglycosylation. It is not absorbed by the gut and is therefore used to sterilize the gut.

89. (C) Erythromycin.
A macrolide such as erythromycin does not increase the risk of nephrotoxicity. However, it increases the risk for skin rashes, GI distress, eosinophilia, hepatitis and inhibition of CYP450 enzymes that metabolize drugs like digoxin, carbamazepine and theophylline.

90. (B) Echinocandins.
Echinocandins drugs inhibit the synthesis of β (1-3)-glucan used for making the cell walls of fungi. They do not affect the permeability of the cell membrane. Side effects associated with its infusion include fever, rashes, GI distress and flushing.

Test 6: Questions

1. Which of the following antifungals blocks the functions of microtubules of fungi?
   A. Terbinafine
   B. Echinocandins
   C. Flucytosine
   D. Griseofulvin

2. Michael is scheduled to have an amphotericin B infusion. He must be premedicated with all except which of the following?
   A. Antihistamines
   B. Antipyretics
   C. Vitamin B6
   D. Glucocorticoids

3. All except which of the following statements are correct about griseofulvin?
   A. It is active in its topical form.
   B. It is contraindicated in patients with porphyria.
   C. It is fungistatic.
   D. It activates the hepatic metabolism of warfarin.

4. Which of the following azoles has the highest risk for drug-drug interactions?
   A. Fluconazole
   B. Ketoconazole
   C. Itraconazole
   D. Voriconazole

5. Which of the following antifungals is nephrotoxic?
   A. Flucytosine
   B. Ketoconazole
   C. Terbinafine
   D. Griseofulvin

6. All except which of the following antiviral drugs are used to treat herpes?
   A. Acyclovir
   B. Abacavir
   C. Ganciclovir
   D. Foscarnet

7. All except which of the following are examples of nucleoside reverse transcriptase inhibitors?
   A. Lamivudine
   B. Zidovudine
   C. Efavirenz
   D. Emtricitabine

8. Which of the following is not a protease inhibitor?
   A. Tenofovir
   B. Indinavir
   C. Atazanavir
   D. Darunavir

9. Which of the following is an entry and fusion inhibitor?
   A. Oseltamivir
   B. Nevirapine
   C. Maraviroc
   D. Amantadine

10. Which of the following drugs is used to treat hepatitis?
   A. Ribavirin
   B. Oseltamivir
   C. Zanamivir
   D. Etravirine

11. Which of the following statements is false about metronidazole?
    A. It is effective against anaerobic infections.
    B. Its use increases the risk for pseudomembranous colitis.
    C. It causes a disulfiram-like effect if taken with alcohol.
    D. It can block the metabolism of warfarin.

12. Which of the following is not a urinary antiseptic?
    A. Nalidixic acid
    B. Polymyxin
    C. Nitrofurantoin
    D. Methenamine

13. Which of the following letters is not a Roman numeral?
    A. X
    B. B
    C. D
    D. I

14. Which of the following Roman numerals represents the number 15?
    A. XIV
    B. XX
    C. VX
    D. XV

15. Which of the following medical abbreviations is incorrectly paired?
    A. LA – Less acting
    B. SR – Sustained release
    C. CR – Controlled release
    D. DS – Double strength

16. Which of the following does not describe the trade name of a medication?
    A. It is also known as the proprietary name.
    B. It is usually the most prominent name on the drug label.
    C. It refers to the name given to a medication by its manufacturer.
    D. It is also known as the nonproprietary name.

17. Which of the following statements is false regarding dosage strength?
   A. It refers to the amount of the drug contained in a specific unit of measurement.
   B. It is usually measured in milligrams.
   C. It refers to the full quantity of the drug contained in a bottle.
   D. None of the above.

18. Which of the following is not a method used for the calculation of drug dosages?
   A. Basic formula
   B. Fractional equation
   C. Ratio and proportion
   D. None of the above

19. A physician orders ciprofloxacin 0.5g PO, BID for a patient. The drug available is ciprofloxacin 250 mg. How many tablets should the patient take?
   A. 2
   B. 4
   C. 1
   D. 3

20. A patient is required to take 250 mg of amoxicillin and the dose available is 125 mg/5 mL. Which of these formulas represents the ratio and proportion method of calculating the quantity of drug the patient should take?
   A. On-hand dose: Vehicle = Desired dose : Amount to give
   B. On-hand dose: Amount to give = Desired dose : Vehicle
   C. Desired dose: Vehicle = On-hand dose : Amount to give
   D. None of the above

21. Which of the following factors is not necessary when calculating drug dosages using the dimensional analysis method?
   A. Conversional factor
   B. Drug label factor
   C. Drug order factor
   D. None of the above

22. Disadvantages of oral drug administration include all except which of the following?
   A. Varied rate of drug absorption
   B. Irritation of the gastric mucosa
   C. Less risk of aspiration into the lungs
   D. Discoloration of the tooth enamel

23. A vial of Ceftriaxone contains 1,000 mg. What amount of diluent is to be added to obtain a solution containing 100 mg/mL?
   A. 5 mL
   B. 10 mL
   C. 20 mL
   D. 1 mL

24. Ms. Jones has come to the pharmacy to receive the following medication ordered by her physician: Caps Amoxicillin 500 mg PO QID. The dose of amoxicillin on hand at the pharmacy is 250 mg. How should Ms. Jones take this medication?
   A. 4 capsules taken 2 times each day
   B. 2 capsules, taken 4 times each day
   C. 2 capsules taken every 4 hours
   D. 2 capsules taken once every 4 days

25. James complains of a burning sensation in his epigastric region that is worse when he is hungry. He admits to taking over-the-counter NSAIDS frequently for his knee pain. Which of the following medications will be least useful in treating his condition?
   A. Cimetidine
   B. Omeprazole
   C. Docusate
   D. Bismuth subsalicylate

26. You are to compound 50 mL of a 1:500 solution of diazepam. How many milligrams of this drug are required?

A. 25
B. 250
C. 10
D. 100

27. How many milligrams of ketoconazole are in a 30 mL tube of 5% ketoconazole?

A. 15
B. 0.15
C. 1,500
D. 150

28. How many grams of chloramphenicol are in a 20 g tube of 1% chloramphenicol ointment?

A. 20
B. 1
C. 0.2
D. 200

29. You are to compound 20 g of lactic acid in 1 L of Ringer's lactate. What is the percentage of this solution?

A. 20%
B. 2%
C. 0.2%
D. 200%

30. 500 mL of eucalyptus oil has 5 g of menthol. What is the percentage of this solution?

A. 5%
B. 1%
C. 50%
D. 10%

31. You are compounding 2 g of a solid in 50 mL of liquid. What is the percentage of this solution?

A. 10%

B. 25%

C. 4%

D. 8%

32. A solution has 200 mg/mL. What is the percentage of drugs in this solution?

A. 2%

B. 20%

C. 0.2%

D. 200%

33. How many mg of cortisone is in 5 mL of a 2% cortisone cream?

A. 1

B. 100

C. 10

D. 25

34. You are to infuse 300 mL of fluid in 60 minutes. If your drop factor is 10 gtt/mL, what is the flow rate in gtt/min?

A. 100

B. 50

C. 150

D. 200

35. Which of the following is true about sharps bins?

A. They should be kept in an area without easy access.

B. They must not be easily transported.

C. They should be removed and replaced when three-fourths full.

D. They should never be separated from other containers.

36. All except which of the following antidiabetic drugs increases the risk of hypoglycemia?

A. Insulin
B. Tolbutamide
C. Exenatide
D. Metformin

37. Which of the following is false concerning barcoding?

A. It can be used to tag drug names.
B. It can be used to tag packaging size.
C. It can tag drug dosage form.
D. It cannot track stock level at the register.

38. Which of the following is not information required for a prescription order refill form?

A. Physician's name and address
B. The number of refills
C. The drug dose and form
D. Patient's next of kin

39. Which of the following classes of antidiabetic drugs increase the risk of heart failure?

A. Thiazolidinediones
B. Glucagon-like peptide-1
C. Insulin secretagogues
D. Biguanides

40. All except ____________ are adverse effects of insulin.

A. Hypoglycemia
B. Hyperglycemia
C. Lipodystrophy
D. Somogyi effect

41. Which of the following is a prescription error?
    A. Incorrect drug
    B. Incorrect patient identification
    C. Early refills
    D. All of the above

42. A patient presents to the pharmacy with complaints of receiving a different drug than was prescribed by her physician. Which of the following options is not a step to be taken by the CPhT to avoid a wrong-drug error?
    A. Check the drug when taking it out of the drug container.
    B. Check the drug after placing it on the drug dispenser.
    C. Check the drug before returning it to the container.
    D. Double-check the drug after dispensing it to the patient.

43. Prevention of prescription errors includes __________.
    A. Checking the drug three times.
    B. Double-checking patient identification.
    C. Double-checking abnormal doses.
    D. All of the above.

44. A CPhT receives a prescription order for an OTC cough medication that contains pseudoephedrine. He suspects the patient has forged the prescription of the cough syrup. Which of the following is one way to detect if a patient has forged a prescription?
    A. Check the DEA number.
    B. Check if the prescription is folded.
    C. Call the local police.
    D. Verify with a CPhT supervisor.

45. Which of the following is true concerning the use of a DEA number?
    A. It is used to track the delivery of controlled substances.
    B. The first letter of the DEA number denotes the prescriber's practice.
    C. The second letter of the DEA number is the first letter of the prescriber's last name.
    D. All of the above.

46. Peter has come to the pharmacy complaining of the frequent passage of loose stools since he ate sushi earlier. Which of the following medications will he not benefit from?

A. Sucralfate
B. Loperamide
C. Kaopectate
D. Diphenoxylate

47. Which of the following is not a side effect of omeprazole?

A. Headaches
B. Constipation
C. Flatulence
D. Heartburn

48. Which of the following medications is not indicated in the treatment of a nematode infestation?

A. Pyrantel pamoate
B. Imodium
C. Mebendazole
D. Albendazole

49. Metronidazole is useful in treating all except which of the following infections?

A. Amoebiasis
B. Filariasis
C. Trichomoniasis
D. Giardiasis

50. Which of the following is the drug of choice for treating patients with a nematode infestation?

A. Praziquantel
B. Albendazole
C. Primaquine
D. Ivermectin

51. Which of the following is the drug of choice for treating patients with a tapeworm infestation?

A. Praziquantel
B. Albendazole
C. Primaquine
D. Ivermectin

52. Which of the following is not an alkylating agent?

A. Cyclophosphamide
B. Cisplatin
C. Gemcitabine
D. Busulfan

53. Which of the following chemotherapeutic agents increases the risk of hemorrhagic cystitis?

A. Cyclophosphamide
B. Flucytosine
C. Doxorubicin
D. Busulfan

54. Which of the following drugs inhibits the synthesis of folic acid?

A. Fluorouracil
B. Methotrexate
C. Mercaptopurine
D. Gemcitabine

55. All except which of the following drugs inhibits the synthesis of pyrimidines?

A. Fluorouracil
B. Thioguanine
C. Cytarabine
D. Gemcitabine

56. Which of the following best describes the mechanism of action of vinca alkaloids?

A. They block the formation of mitotic spindles.
B. They block topoisomerase II.
C. They cause intercalation of DNA pairs.
D. They block the synthesis of purines.

57. Which of the following is a podophyllotoxin?

A. Vinblastine
B. Etoposide
C. Paclitaxel
D. Topotecan

58. Which of the following chemotherapeutic agents is specific for cardiotoxicity?

A. Doxorubicin
B. Paclitaxel
C. Etoposide
D. Vincristine

59. Which of the following chemotherapeutic agents is specific for pulmonary fibrosis?

A. Rituximab
B. Doxorubicin
C. Paclitaxel
D. Bleomycin

60. A patient on methotrexate is also treated with levocurin. Which of the following best describes the mechanism of action of leucovorin?

A. It binds to the metabolite of methotrexate in the kidneys.
B. It binds to the metabolite of methotrexate in the liver.
C. It rescues red blood cells.
D. It replenishes DHFR.

61. A patient on fluorouracil is also treated with leucovorin. Which of the following best describes the mechanism of action of leucovorin?

A. It binds to the metabolite of methotrexate in the kidneys.
B. It binds to the metabolite of methotrexate in the liver.
C. It potentiates the action of fluorouracil.
D. It inhibits the metabolism of fluorouracil.

62. Which of the following statements is false about telephone orders for controlled substances?

A. Pharmacies may ordinarily accept telephone orders for medications in Schedules II, III, IV and V.
B. Practitioners prescribing Schedule II medications for long-term care facilities may transmit the prescription via a facsimile to a dispensing pharmacy.
C. An oral order may be allowed for Schedule II substances in emergencies.
D. A facsimile may be considered as a written prescription in some situations.

63. Which of the following schedules of medications may not be filled via electronic prescription?

A. II
B. III
C. IV
D. I

64. Concerning partial refills of Schedules III, IV and V drugs, which of the following statements does not meet the DEA guidelines?

A. Each partial refill must be just as a refill.
B. The total amount of medications dispensed in partial refills is the same as the total quantity prescribed.
C. No dispensing occurs beyond the established limit for the drug, depending on the drug schedule.
D. None of the above.

65. When storing hazardous drugs, which of the following does not apply?

A. They should be stored on a separate shelf at or below eye level.
B. Labels on these drugs should alert workers of their potentially hazardous nature.
C. PPE should be worn when receiving and storing hazardous drugs.
D. Volatile substances should be placed in an airtight environment.

66. Concerning recordkeeping for controlled drugs, which of the following information is untrue?

A. Records must be maintained for two years.
B. Records for Schedules II and III drugs only must be kept separate from records and inventories of other drugs.
C. A notation must be used to distinguish controlled substances from other medications.
D. Records of scheduled drugs are required to be readily retrievable.

67. Inventory requirements for controlled substances include all except which of the following?

A. The DEA requires pharmacies to take inventory of controlled substances every two years.
B. Each pharmacy is mandated to submit an inventory of controlled substances biannually.
C. Estimated counts may be used for inventory of Schedule III, IV and V substances.
D. Actual counts should be done when taking inventory of Schedule II substances.

68. Which of the following statements about controlled substances is untrue?

A. Some states may differ in their practices in regards to regulations for controlled substances.
B. The DEA allows the transfer of original prescription information for Schedules III and IV drugs.
C. A DEA number consists of two letters and five digits.
D. Controlled medications may be stored in a secure vault or dispersed throughout the pharmacy stock.

69. Which of the following statements is correct about handling hazardous substances?

A. It is necessary to carry Material Safety Data Sheets for all hazardous substances on all premises where they are handled.
B. Segregating inventories into drug categories may help prevent harmful errors.
C. Hazardous drugs should be placed in a sealed, protective outer bag to contain spills in case their container leaks or breaks.
D. All of the above.

70. Which of the following steps is not necessary to perform when a controlled substance is stolen?

A. Fill out and file DEA Form 106.
B. Contact the DEA and local police.
C. Report all thefts within 24 hours.
D. None of the above.

71. Which of the following is not a disease-modifying antirheumatic drug?

A. Aspirin
B. Leflunomide
C. Methotrexate
D. Hydroxychloroquine

72. Joe, a 55-year-old male, is being managed with colchicine for gouty arthritis. Which of the following describes the mechanism of action of this drug?

A. Blocks reabsorption of uric acid
B. Prevents release of inflammatory mediators
C. Blocks leukocyte migration
D. Blocks breakdown of xanthine to uric acid

73. Which of the following drugs prevents the reabsorption of uric acid?
   A. Probenecid
   B. Allopurinol
   C. Colchicine
   D. Uricase

74. Which of the following best describes the mechanism of action of allopurinol?
   A. Blocks reabsorption of uric acid
   B. Prevents release of inflammatory mediators
   C. Blocks leukocyte migration
   D. Blocks breakdown of xanthine to uric acid

75. Which of the following drugs is suitable for use in an 80-year-old female with fecal impaction and a history of oral opioids for chronic back pain?
   A. Lactulose
   B. Bisacodyl
   C. Phosphate enema
   D. Omeprazole

76. Which of the following is the drug of choice for chlamydia?
   A. Vancomycin
   B. Doxycycline
   C. Metronidazole
   D. Ciprofloxacin

77. Which of the following drugs for gout is likely to increase serum concentrations of methotrexate?
   A. Probenecid
   B. Allopurinol
   C. Colchicine
   D. Aspirin

78. Ferb is a 45-year-old male on nicotinic for dyslipidemia. He will probably experience which of the following symptoms?

A. Bloating
B. Peripheral neuropathy
C. Flushing
D. Headaches

79. Which of the following is the mechanism of action of cholestyramine?

A. Inhibits cholesterol synthesis
B. Inhibits gut absorption of cholesterol
C. Inhibits lipid transporters in the gut
D. Stimulates oxidation of fatty acids

80. Which of the following antilipid agents decreases the absorption of vitamin K?

A. Atorvastatin
B. Colestipol
C. Ezetimibe
D. Nicotinic acid

81. Which of the following is a major adverse effect of gemfibrozil?

A. Constipation
B. Hyperuricemia
C. Cholelithiasis
D. Steatorrhea

82. Substances that are yet to be approved for human use by the FDA but are used in clinical trials are called ______________.

A. Controlled substances
B. Investigational drugs
C. Chemotherapeutic agents
D. Over-the-counter medications

83. Which of the following is true concerning investigational drugs?
A. They have FDA approval.
B. They are available only for patients who are terminally ill.
C. The unused portion must be returned to the provider on expiration or drug discontinuation.
D. They must be kept with other drugs in the pharmacy.

84. Which of the following controlled substances has the least potential for abuse?
A. Schedule I
B. Schedule II
C. Schedule V
D. Schedule III

85. A patient was prescribed amoxicillin tablets for the treatment of an upper respiratory tract infection. She approaches the CPhT with her prescription. The prescribed antibiotics have an automatic stop date of ___________.
A. 7 days
B. 5 days
C. 14 days
D. Determined by the prescribing physician

86. Ned, a CPhT, received a prescription order for Valium. What is the maximum amount of refills that can be given for Valium?
A. Twice a month refill
B. No refills, as it is a controlled substance
C. Five refills in six months from the date of prescription
D. As often as patient and subscriber agree

87. A new CPhT receives a prescription order for a Schedule II medication. A Schedule II prescription order has a maximum amount of how many refills?
A. Five in six months
B. As often as patient and prescriber agree
C. None
D. Three in a year

88. Which of the following groups of patients would benefit from brightly colored stickers used to differentiate their medication?

A. Visually impaired individuals
B. Elderly patients
C. Hearing-impaired individuals
D. Patients of different cultural backgrounds and ethnicity

89. The pharmacy receives an order for a 20-day supply of Lasix 20 mg to be taken three times a day. The pharmacy has in stock 10 mg Lasix tablets. How many tablets must the CPhT prepare for a 20-day supply?

A. 50
B. 100
C. 200
D. 120

90. Which of the following is a selective alpha 1 adrenergic receptor blocker?

A. Phentolamine
B. Prazosin
C. Yohimbine
D. Butoxamine

Test 6: Answers and Explanations

1. (D) Griseofulvin.
Griseofulvin inhibits the synthesis of nucleic acid and disrupts microtubular function. It is fungistatic. Side effects include headaches, GI distress, photosensitivity, confusion and elevated liver enzymes. It causes a disulfiram-like effect with alcohol and decreases the serum concentrations of warfarin.

2. (C) Vitamin B6.
Michael does not need to be premedicated with Vitamin B6. Side effects associated with the infusion of amphotericin B include chills, fever, vomiting and hypotension. To prevent this from occurring, the drug should be infused slowly. Also, antipyretics, antihistamines and glucocorticoids should be given before the infusion. Other side effects include renal tubular acidosis, anemia and neurotoxicity.

3. (A) It is active in its topical form.
This statement is false because griseofulvin is not active in its topical form. It is available only as an oral drug.

4. (B) Ketoconazole.
Ketoconazole inhibits the metabolism of warfarin, phenytoin oral hypoglycemics and cyclosporine and has the highest risk for drug-drug interactions. It also increases the risk for infertility, gynecomastia and menstrual abnormalities. For these reasons, parenteral forms are unavailable in the United States.

5. (A) Flucytosine.
Flucytosine and amphotericin B are nephrotoxic antifungal drugs. Azoles, terbinafine and griseofulvin increase the risk of hepatitis and deranged hepatic enzymes.

6. (B) Abacavir.

This is a nucleoside reverse transcriptase inhibitor used to treat HIV, not herpes.

7. (C) Efavirenz.
Efavirenz is a nonnucleoside reverse transcriptase inhibitor used to treat HIV.

8. (A) Tenofovir.
Tenofovir is not a protease inhibitor. It's a nucleoside reverse transcriptase inhibitor.

9. (C) Maraviroc.
Maraviroc and enfuvirtide are entry and fusion inhibitors.

10. (A) Ribavirin.
Ribavirin is used to treat infectious hepatitis. Other drugs used include IFN-α, adefovir dipivoxil and entecavir.

11. (B) Its use increases the risk for pseudomembranous colitis.
This statement is false because metronidazole is an effective treatment against pseudomembranous colitis. Its use, however, increases the risk for opportunistic fungal infections.

12. (B) Polymyxin.
Polymyxin is not a urinary antiseptic. Urinary antiseptics are used to sterilize the bladder because they are quickly excreted via the urine. Since they are negligibly absorbed into the systemic circulation, they exert their effect on the bladder. Examples include nalidixic acid, nitrofurantoin and methenamine.

13. (B) B.
B is not a Roman numeral. The Roman numerals are built around seven letters: I, V, X, L, C, D and M. Roman numerals are used less commonly than Arabic numbers in dosage calculations. However, some practitioners still use this system in prescriptions, so it is necessary for the CPhT to understand Roman numerals.

14. (D) XV.
In Roman numerals, 10 is written as X, and 5 is written as V, so 15 is written as X and V.

15. (A) LA – Less acting.
This is incorrectly paired. LA is the abbreviation for *long-acting*. These kinds of medications are slowly absorbed after they are administered and their effects last a long time.

16. (D) It is also known as the nonproprietary name.
A medication's trade name refers to the name given to the drug by the manufacturer. It is also called the brand or proprietary name and is usually the most prominent name printed on a drug label, often followed by the trademark symbol, which indicates that the name of the medication and its formulation is registered.

17. (C) It refers to the full quantity of the drug contained in a bottle.
This is false. The dosage strength of a medication refers to its dosage weight, that is, the amount of the drug provided in a specific unit of measurement. Usually, medications are measured in milligrams, but some drugs may come in two different but equivalent dosage strengths, such as "milligrams per tablet" and "units per tablet."

18. (D) None of the above.
Drug dosages can be calculated using four methods: basic formula, fractional equation, ratio and proportion and dimensional analysis. These methods are commonly used by technicians or pharmacists when calculating the dose of a drug becomes necessary.

19. (A) 2.
To convert from milligrams to grams, move the decimal points three spaces to the right or multiply by 1,000.
0.5 g = 500 mg

Using the basic formula:

D/H x V
Where D = Dosage ordered
H = The dose available (that is, the drug dose on the label of the container)
V = The form in which the drug is supplied (tablet, capsule, suspension, etc.)

So, (500/250) x 1 = 2 tablets.

20. (A) On-hand dose : Vehicle = Desired dose : Amount to give.
The ratio and proportion method is the oldest method used to calculate dosages. The formula is as follows:
On-hand dose: Vehicle = Desired dose : Amount to give
The inner values in this formula are known as the means, while the outer values are known as the extremes.

21. (D) None of the above.
The dimensional analysis method is also known as the label factor method and is used for calculating dosages with three factors: drug label, drug order and conversional factors.

22. (C) Less risk of aspiration into the lungs.
Disadvantages of oral drug administration do not include less risk of aspiration into the lungs. Taking medications by mouth poses an increased risk of aspiration into the lungs, compared to the parenteral route. Other disadvantages include the destruction of the drugs by the digestive enzymes, leading to their reduced bioavailability and increased chance of liver retention of the drug, leading to liver diseases.

23. (B) 10 mL.
Using the rate and ratio method of calculation:
100 :1 mL = 1,000: X
X = 1,000/100
X = 10 mL

24. (B) 2 capsules, taken 4 times each day.

Ms. Jones should take two capsules of amoxicillin four times each day, by mouth.

25. (C) Docusate.
Docusate will be least useful in treating this condition. It is a stool softener used to treat occasional constipation. It works by increasing the absorption of water the stool absorbs from the gut, thereby making the stool softer. Cimetidine is a type 2 histamine receptor blocker, while omeprazole is a proton pump inhibitor. These drugs, together with bismuth subsalicylate (a coating agent), are useful in the treatment of gastrointestinal ulcers.

26. (D) 100.
1:500 = 1 g/500 mL
1 g/500 mL = X g/50 mL

X g = 50 mL × 1 g/500 mL
X = 0.1 g = 100 mg

27. (C) 1,500.
5% solution = 5 g/100 mL
5 g/100 mL = X g/30 mL

X g = 30 mL × 5 g/100 mL
X = 1.5 g = 1.500 mg

28. (C) 0.2.
1% weight = 1 g/100 g
1 g/100 g = X g/20 g

X g = 1 g × 20 g/100 mg

X = 0.2 g

29. (B) 2%.
First, convert liters to milliliters = 1,000 mL.

20 g/1,000 mL = 2 g/100 mL = 2% solution.

30. (B) 1%.
5 g/500 mL = 1 g/100 mL = 1%.

31. (D) 8%.
2 g/50 mL = 2 g × 2/50 mL × 2 = 4 g/100 mL = 4%.

32. (B) 20%.
Convert 200 mg to grams = 0.2 g/mL.

0.2 g × 100 / 1 mL× 100 = 20 g/100 mL = 20%.

33. (B) 100.
2% = 2 g/100 mL
2 g/100 mL = X g/5 mL
X g = 2 g × 5 mL/100 mL

X = 0.1 g = 100 mg.

34. (B) 50.
Drops per minute = [Total IV volume/Time (minute)] X Drop Factor

Drops per minute = X
Drop factor = 10 gtt/mL
V = 300 mL
Time = 60 minutes

X = (300/60) × 10 gtt/mL
X = 50 gtt/min

35. (C) They should be removed and replaced when three-fourths full.
To ensure work safety, a sharps container should be placed in an area where the staff can have easy access to it. It should be easily transported, be removed

and replaced when nearly full and should be kept separated from other containers.

36. (D) Metformin.
Metformin is a biguanide. It blocks renal and hepatic gluconeogenesis and stimulates glycolysis in peripheral tissues. It does not cause hypoglycemia. Side effects include gastrointestinal symptoms like diarrhea and nausea, and lactic acidosis, particularly in alcoholic patients and patients with liver or renal disease.

37. (D) It cannot track stock level at the register.
This is false. Barcoding can provide information on the drug name, package size, dosage form, strength, dose and quantity of the drug. It can be used to track the stock level at the register.

38. (D) Patient's next of kin.
The information required on a prescription order refill form includes the physician's name and address, number of refills, drug dose and form, patient's insurance or medical record, physician signature and DEA number. Information on the patient's next of kin is not necessary.

39. (A) Thiazolidinediones.
These drugs increase tissue sensitivity to insulin by stimulating the peroxisome proliferator–activated receptor-gamma nuclear receptor (PPAR-f receptor). Side effects include heart failure, edema and anemia.

40. (B) Hyperglycemia.
Hyperglycemia is not an adverse effect of insulin. The adverse effects of insulin include hypoglycemia, insulin lipodystrophy and Somogyi effect. The Somogyi effect causes periods of hypoglycemia followed by rebound hyperglycemia, which often occurs after the administration of insulin.

41. (D) All of the above.

Prescription errors include incorrect drugs, incorrect patient identification, early refills, wrong drug strength, forged drug orders and abnormal doses. Hence, the CPhT must be mindful to prevent this error.

42. (D) Double-check the drug after dispensing it to the patient.
To avoid a wrong-drug error, the medication should be checked three times. Check the drug when taking it out from the drug container, after placing it on the drug dispenser, and before returning it to the drug container. These steps help prevent the technician from dispensing the wrong drug to the patient.

43. (D) All of the above.
To prevent prescription errors, check the drug three times, double-check the patient's identification to be sure it matches the patient, double-check abnormal doses and make sure to retrieve the right drug dose. Route and time to take the medication should also be verified.

44. (A) Check the DEA number.
The DEA registration number is used to track the prescription of controlled substances. Other means of identifying a forged prescription include checking the indication of the prescription against those that are found on the package insert of the drug, checking patient identification, double-checking handwritten orders and remaining vigilant on the number of prescriptions by a particular prescriber.

45. (D) All of the above.
The DEA number is a registration number that appears on every prescription. It enables tracking of controlled substances. The first letter of the DEA number denotes the prescriber's practice. The second letter of the DEA number is the first letter of the prescriber's name.

46. (A) Sucralfate.
Peter will not benefit from sucralfate. Sucralfate is an antacid medication that acts by forming a protective coat over gastrointestinal ulcers by binding to the ulcer base, thereby allowing them to heal. It is not useful as an antidiarrheal agent.

47. (D) Heartburn.
Heartburn is not a side effect of omeprazole. Omeprazole is a proton pump inhibitor used in the management of gastrointestinal ulcers and reflux disease. It works by inhibiting proton pumps in the gastrointestinal mucosa, thereby reducing the production of gastric acid. Side effects of this medication include headache, constipation, diarrhea or vomiting and flatulence. Serious side effects are rare and include liver damage and subacute cutaneous lupus erythematosus.

48. (B) Imodium.
Imodium is not indicated in the treatment of nematode infections. Nematodes and other parasites can easily be picked up by children from soil or infected pets and anthelmintics are used in the treatment of these parasites. They include mebendazole, thiabendazole and pyrantel pamoate. These drugs act on nematode proteins called tubulin (or enzymes related to the tubulin process), thereby causing paralysis of the organism so that it cannot survive or breed.

49. (B) Filariasis.
Metronidazole is not useful in treating filariasis, which is a disease caused by parasitic worms. Pharmaceutical options include albendazole and ivermectin.

50. (B) Albendazole.
Albendazole is the drug of choice in the treatment of patients with nematode infestation.

51. (A) Praziquantel.
Praziquantel is the drug of choice in treating patients with infestations with trematodes (flukes) and cestodes (tapeworms).

52. (C) Gemcitabine.
This is an antimetabolite. Alkylating agents cause the breakage of DNA strands by alkylating the nucleophilic groups in the bases of DNA. Examples

are cyclophosphamide, mechlorethamine, platinum analogs, busulfan, dacarbazine and procarbazine.

53. (A) Cyclophosphamide.
Cyclophosphamide increases the risk of hemorrhagic cystitis. Premedication with mesna reduces the risk. Other side effects include GI distress, alopecia, myelosuppression, SIADH and pulmonary toxicity.

54. (B) Methotrexate.
Methotrexate inhibits the synthesis of folic acid, while mercaptopurine and thioguanine inhibit the synthesis of purines. Gemcitabine, fluorouracil and cytarabine inhibit the synthesis of pyrimidines.

55. (B) Thioguanine.
Thioguanine inhibits the synthesis of purines, not pyrimidines.

56. (A) They block the formation of mitotic spindles.
Vinca alkaloids inhibit the formation of mitotic spindles. Examples are vincristine, vinblastine and vinorelbine. Side effects include GI distress, bone marrow suppression and alopecia.

57. (B) Etoposide.
Podophyllotoxins include teniposide and etoposide. They stimulate the breakage of DNA strands by blocking topoisomerase II. Side effects include GI distress and bone marrow suppression.

58. (A) Doxorubicin.
Cardiotoxicity is peculiar to the anthracyclines (epirubicin, doxorubicin, daunorubicin and mitoxantrone). They block the action of topoisomerase II and cause the intercalation of DNA pairs.

59. (D) Bleomycin.
This drug is specific for pulmonary fibrosis. Other side effects include hypersensitivity reactions, alopecia, hyperkeratosis and blisters.

60. (D) It replenishes DHFR.
Methotrexate is an antimetabolite that blocks the action of dihydrofolate reductase (DHFR). Leucovorin is the reduced form of folic acid that replenishes DHFR in normal cells.

61. (C) It potentiates the action of fluorouracil.
Leucovorin potentiates the action of fluorouracil by stimulating the release of cofactors and decreasing the synthesis of thymidine. These actions allow lower doses of fluorouracil to be safely administered to the patient.

62. (A) Pharmacies may ordinarily accept telephone orders for medications in Schedules II, III, IV and V.
This is false. Under ordinary circumstances, Schedule II prescriptions may not be made over the phone or via a fax machine. However, the DEA allows for exceptional situations where telephone prescription of Schedule II medication may be allowed.

63. (D) I.
Schedule I medications may not be filled via electronic prescription. Pharmacies and physicians are allowed to transmit prescriptions for Schedules II, III, IV and V drugs, provided they are using properly certified software (that is, SureScripts). While this change occurred in federal law as of June 1, 2010, some states may still not allow e-prescription for controlled substances.

64. (D) None of the above.
All the above are correct. The federal regulations code states that the partial refill of a prescription for controlled substances is allowed, as long as each partial refill is recorded in the same manner as a refilling, the total amount of drugs dispensed in partial fills does not surpass the total amount prescribed and dispensing occurs for not more than six months for Schedules III and IV medications and not more than 12 months for Schedule V medications.

65. (D) Volatile substances should be placed in an airtight environment.

This does not apply to hazardous drugs. Volatile or flammable substances, such as tax-free alcohol, require careful storage. These items should be placed in a cool location with proper ventilation. They should be stored in an area designed to reduce the chances of explosion or fire outbreak.

66. (B) Records for Schedules II and III drugs only must be kept separate from records and inventories of other drugs.
This is untrue. Each pharmacy must keep an accurate record of every controlled substance that is received, dispensed or disposed of. It is required that inventory for Schedules II to IV drugs be kept differently from the inventory of other medications. However, this information should be readily retrievable and be maintained for two years. It is important to distinguish controlled drugs from other items with some notations or other visually identifiable marks, for example, a red line or an asterisk.

67. (B) Each pharmacy is mandated to submit an inventory of controlled substances biannually.
While the DEA mandates every pharmacy to take an inventory of controlled substances biannually, submission of an inventory record is not required unless requested by the DEA.

68. (C) A DEA number consists of two letters and five digits.
This is untrue. A DEA number is a series of numbers assigned to health-care providers that allows them to write prescriptions for controlled substances. It consists of two letters and seven digits.

69. (D) All of the above.
OSHA requires all workplaces to possess MSDS for all hazardous substances that are stored on their premises. The MSDS contains information about handling, cleanup and first aid when dealing with these substances.

70. (D) None of the above.
In the event that a controlled substance is stolen or found to be missing from a pharmacy, the pharmacy should contact the local police and the DEA. Reports should be made within 24 hours, as required by the DEA. It is also necessary

to fill out a DEA Form 106. This form can be filed electronically or in hard copy.

71. (A) Aspirin.
Aspirin is not a disease-modifying antirheumatic drug because it does not slow down inflammatory changes in the joints. However, aspirin is used to manage chronic pain in patients with rheumatoid arthritis.

72. (C) Blocks leukocyte migration.
Colchicine blocks the aggregation of microtubules necessary for the migration of leukocytes and phagocytosis.

73. (A) Probenecid.
Probenecid is a uricosuric drug that prevents the reabsorption of uric acid. This action increases the excretion of uric acid. Another drug that does this is sulfinpyrazone.

74. (D) Blocks breakdown of xanthine to uric acid.
Allopurinol inhibits xanthine oxidase, an enzyme that metabolizes hypoxanthine to xanthine and then to uric acid.

75. (C) Phosphate enema.
A phosphate enema is the best choice for fecal impaction, not an oral laxative or stool softener. Laxatives can increase the risk of intestinal rupture. Omeprazole is of no use in this case.

76. (B) Doxycycline.
The treatment of uncomplicated chlamydia trachomatis includes a single dose of azithromycin or doxycycline given twice daily for seven days, erythromycin given for seven days, or ofloxacin or levofloxacin each given for seven days.

77. (A) Probenecid.
Probenecid will compete with methotrexate for reabsorption at the proximal tubule because methotrexate is also a weak acid. Since methotrexate will not be excreted, serum concentrations will rise.

78. (C) Flushing.
Nicotinic acid is used to reduce serum concentrations of LDL and VLDL and increase serum concentrations of HDL. The most common adverse effect is flushing, which can be prevented by pretreatment with an NSAID. Other side effects include itching and vomiting.

79. (B) Inhibits gut absorption of cholesterol.
Cholestyramine is a resin that binds to bile and prevents its absorption into the enterohepatic circulation. A side effect of this inhibition is that it prevents absorption of fat-soluble vitamins like vitamin K; thiazides and warfarin; and dietary folic acid.

80. (B) Colestipol.
Colestipol is a resin that binds to bile and prevents its absorption into the enterohepatic circulation. A side effect of this inhibition is that it prevents absorption of fat-soluble vitamins like vitamin K, thiazides and warfarin, and dietary folic acid.

81. (C) Cholelithiasis.
Side effects of gemfibrozil include cholelithiasis, nausea, skin rashes and reduced white blood cell and red blood cell count.

82. (B) Investigational drugs.
Investigational drugs are yet to be approved by the FDA for use in humans. These drugs are used in clinical trials and may be dispensed only under special circumstances. Controlled substances are drugs that require a prescription before they can be dispensed. Over-the-counter medications do not require prescriptions.

83. (C) The unused portions must be returned to the provider on expiration or drug discontinuation.
This is true. Investigational drugs are not FDA approved. They should be kept separate from other drugs in the pharmacy, and unused portions must be returned to the provider on expiration or drug discontinuation. They are

dispensed only under special circumstances when prescribed by a physician after getting due permission from the sponsor. Each patient on an investigational drug must have their supply.

84. (C) Schedule V.
Schedule V substances have limited potential for abuse. They include small amounts of narcotics, such as codeine used in antitussive and antidiarrheal medication. Schedules I and II have a high potential for abuse and Schedule III has a high tendency for physical or psychological dependence.

85. (C) 14 days.
Antibiotics have an automatic stop date of 14 days. This helps reduce the incidence of antibiotic drug resistance. Nonadherence to antibiotic medication has been linked to a higher incidence of antibiotic resistance.

86. (C) Five refills in six months from the date of the prescription.
Valium is a Schedule IV controlled substance and has the potential for physical and psychological dependence. The maximum amount of refills for Schedule IV substances is five refills in six months from the date of the prescription.

87. (C) None.
Schedule II drugs carry severe restrictions and have no refills. They have a very high potential for abuse with severe physical and psychological dependence. Schedule II drug prescriptions cannot be transferred between pharmacies, and dispensing this group of drugs requires a written prescription.

88. (A) Visually impaired individuals.
Brightly colored stickers can help visually impaired patients identify their medication.

89. (D) 120.
The dosage strength of Lasix in stock = 10 mg.
Requested dose = 20 mg three times daily

2 tabs of 10 mg Lasix = 1 tab of Lasix 20 mg
2 tabs of Lasix X 3 times daily = 6 tabs of 10 mg Lasix daily
For 20 days = 6 tabs of Lasix 10 mg x 20 days= 120 tablets of 10 mg Lasix.

90. (B) Prazosin.
Irreversible nonselective blockers include phenoxybenzamine. Reversible nonselective blockers include phentolamine. Selective alpha 1 blockers include prazosin. Selective alpha 2 blockers include yohimbine. Nonselective beta-blockers include propranolol. Beta 1 blockers include atenolol. Beta 2 blockers include butoxamine.

Made in United States
North Haven, CT
06 October 2023

42450346R00226